Oral Cytology

Ravi Mehrotra
Editor

Oral Cytology

A Concise Guide

Springer

Editor
Ravi Mehrotra, MD, PhD, MIAC, FRCPath
Institute of Cytology and Preventive Oncology (ICPO)
Noida - 201301, Uttar Pradesh, India

ISBN 978-1-4614-5220-1 ISBN 978-1-4614-5221-8 (eBook)
DOI 10.1007/978-1-4614-5221-8
Springer New York Heidelberg Dordrecht London

Library of Congress Control Number: 2012951676

Printed on acid-free paper

Springer is part of Springer Science+Business Media (www.springer.com)

Foreword

Oral cancer is a major public health problem all over the world but particularly in the Indian subcontinent. With well-known risk factors—tobacco and alcohol—and the potential for screening, effective measures for prevention and control are warranted.

Cytological examination is a well-established and effective method of screening for cervical cancer, and significant gains have been made in the control of this form of cancer by the routine use of exfoliative cytology. Application of cytology in the oral cavity is not common but it could be used for screening of patients with suspicious premalignant and malignant conditions of the oral cavity. Hence this monograph, designed to provide a state-of-the-art review of the major issues specific to the field of oral cytology, is very timely. This book provides a comprehensive review of all aspects of oral cytology including sample collection, manual/automated analysis, pitfalls, gray zones, and controversies in diagnosis. Ancillary techniques such as DNA ploidy, molecular biology, and biomarkers are also discussed. The book is extensively illustrated with excellent cytological images.

This book will fill a critical need for reliable knowledge on oral cytology and will be useful for pathologists currently in training as well as pathologists and clinicians dealing with the diagnosis of oral lesions. The editors and authors are to be commended for this effort, since it fills an important gap in our current knowledge.

Chicago, IL, USA

Vinay Kumar
Donald N. Pritzker
Professor and Chairman
Department of Pathology,
Biologic Sciences Division
and the Pritzker School of Medicine
University of Chicago

Acknowledgements

The goal of this book is to form a blend between new and existing information about oral cytopathology. It will hopefully serve as a bench-side companion to the general cytopathologist, oral pathologist, specialist in oral medicine, and head and neck experts.

This compendium is a combined effort from authors of different specialties including cytopathologists, oral pathologists, and basic scientists—all of whom have in common an interest in the diagnosis of oral cancer. Experts from four different continents viz. Asia, Africa, Europe, and the Americas have contributed their vast knowledge and experiences in this field.

Acknowledgments are due to my source of inspiration my beloved; my wife, Deepa Mehrotra, my children, Aditi, Shayak and Vinayak; and my well-wishers, especially my teachers/mentors, Drs. Mamta Singh and Premala A. Singh, Allahabad. They are also due to my colleagues, Drs. Vatsala Misra, Kachnar Verma, Vishal Dhingra, Pallavi Singh, and Anshul Singh of the Department of Pathology, Moti Lal Nehru Medical College, Allahabad; Dr. R. Khanna, Allahabad; Drs. V.L. Lahiri and Atul Gupta, Agra; Drs. Raj Mehrotra and M.M. Goel, Lucknow; Col. S.K.P. Matwanakar, Pune; Dr. Maqsood Siddiqi, Kolkatta; Dr. Bernard Fitzharris, Christchurch; Dr. Raj K. Gupta, Wellington, New Zealand; Dr. Svante Orell, Adelaide, Australia; Dr. Bernard Fox, Portland; Dr. Raj Puri, Bethesda; Dr. Vinod B. Shidham, Detroit; Dr. Prabodh Gupta, Philadelphia; Dr. Carlos Bedrossian, Chicago; Dr. Kamlesh Asotra, California; Dr. Rajesh Sharan, Shillong; my numerous MD and Ph.D students around the world including Madhu, Neeta, Anurag, Mayank, Sanjay, Smita, Santosh, Shruti, Ajay, and Rahela; and, of course, the greatest teacher any doctor can possibly have—my patients.

I have special word of thanks to Prof. Vinay Kumar, Chicago Editor-in Chief, Robbins Pathologic Basis of Disease (which provided my first introduction to this fascinating field and help motivate me to embark on this journey) for kindly agreeing to write the preface.

This book is dedicated to my respected mother, Raj Rani Mehrotra and to the fond memory of my father Prof. T.N. Mehrotra, MD, Ph.D. Founder Professor of Pathology and Principal, Moti Lal Nehru Medical College, Allahabad, without whose inspiration and constant guidance, this book would never have seen the light of the day. Finally, grateful thanks are due to the ever-helpful and dynamic team at Springer, especially Richard Hruska, Senior Editor, Clinical Medicine, William Loob, Development Editor, Andy Kwan, Assistant Editor and Maria Luz Calibo, Project Officer without whose support, this monograph would never have seen the light of the day.

Noida, UP, India Ravi Mehrotra, MD, PhD, MIAC, FRCPath

Contents

Contributors

Til Aach Institute of Image Analysis and Computer Vision, RWTH Aachen University, Aachen, Germany

Amir Afrogheh TBH Laboratories, Oral & Maxillofacial Pathology, National Health Laboratory Service, University of the Western Cape, Cape Town, South Africa

André Bell Institute of Image Analysis and Computer Vision, RWTH Aachen University, Aachen, Germany

Leonid Berynskyy Institute of Cytopathology, Heinrich-Heine-University, Düsseldorf, Germany

Stefan Biesterfeld Institute of Cytopathology, Heinrich-Heine-University, Düsseldorf, Germany

Alfred Böcking Institute of Pathology, City-Hospital Düren, Düren, Germany

Deborah J. Carroll Oral CDx Laboratories, Suffern, NY, USA

Vishal Dhingra Department of Pathology, Moti Lal Nehru Medical College, Allahabad, Uttar Pradesh, India

David Friedrich Institute of Image Analysis and Computer Vision, RWTH Aachen University, Aachen, Germany

Sergio Gandolfo Department of Clinical and Biological Sciences, Oral Medicine and Oncology Section, University of Turin, Orbassano, Italy

Jörg Handschel Department of Cranio- and Maxillofacial Surgery, Heinrich-Heine-University, Düsseldorf, Germany

Jos Hille TBH Laboratories, Oral & Maxillofacial Pathology, National Health Laboratory Service, University of the Western Cape, Cape Town, South Africa

Rahela Ibrahim Department of Pathology, Moti Lal Nehru Medical College, Allahabad, Uttar Pradesh, India

Chen Jin Motic China Company, Xiamen, People's Republic of China

Ravi Mehrotra Institute of Cytology and Preventive Oncology (ICPO), Noida, Uttar Pradesh, India

Dietrich Meyer-Ebrecht Institute of Image Analysis and Computer Vision, RWTH Aachen University, Aachen, Germany

Roberto Navone Department of Biomedical Sciences and Human Oncology, Pathology Section, University of Turin, Torino, Italy

Anatomia Patologica, University of Turin, Torino, Italy

Branko Palcic British Columbia Cancer Agency and University of British Columbia, Vancouver, Canada

Monica Pentenero Department of Clinical and Biological Sciences, Oral Medicine and Oral Oncology Section, University of Turin, Orbassano, Italy

Natalia Pomjanski Institute of Cytopathology, Heinrich-Heine-University, Düsseldorf, Germany

Torsten W. Remmerbach Oral Medicine Unit, Department of Oral, Maxillofacial and Facial Plastic Surgery, Leipzig, Germany

Anshul Singh Department of Pathology, Moti Lal Nehru Medical College, Allahabad, Uttar Pradesh, India

Mamta Singh Department of Pathology, Moti Lal Nehru Medical College, Allahabad, Uttar Pradesh, India

Kachnar Varma Department of Pathology, Moti Lal Nehru Medical College, Allahabad, Uttar Pradesh, India

Thomas Würflinger Institute of Image Analysis and Computer Vision, RWTH Aachen University, Aachen, Germany

Richard Yeung Motic China Company, Xiamen, People's Republic of China

Yu Zhang Institute of Image Analysis and Computer Vision, RWTH Aachen University, Aachen, Germany

Chapter 1
Introduction

Ravi Mehrotra

In a recent report from the American Cancer Society, it was estimated that 35,000 new cases of oral cavity and pharyngeal malignancies are likely to be diagnosed in the United States during 2012, and 6,800 patients will die of the disease [1]. Majority of the patients with these lesions are located in developing countries, with the highest prevalence of up to 40% reported in the Indian subcontinent [2]. In developed countries like the United States, the 5 year survival was 63% the period between 1999 and 2005—an increase from 53% during this time period as compared to 1975 and 1977; this difference was found to be statistically significant [1]. The improved survival rates may be partially explained by the increasing use of newer diagnostic modalities that detect the disease in its precursor stage and/or use of newer chemotherapeutic options.

Currently, the most effective way to control oral cancer is to combine early diagnosis and timely as well as appropriate treatment. Because more than 90% of all oral cancers are squamous cell carcinomas, the vast majority of oral cancers will be diagnosed from lesions on the mucosal surfaces.

It is well known that the majority of malignancies, if not all, develop in precancerous fields characterized by specific genetic alterations. Transepithelial "field mapping biopsies" within widespread lesions are even more essential for cytological evaluation and further investigation [3]. Precancerous and cancerous oral lesions may mimic number of benign oral lesions appearing as a white or red lesion (leukoplakia, erythroplakia, and erythro/leukoplakia) [4]. The malignant potential of these lesions is generally assessed by histopathology based on the presence and the degree of dysplasia in biopsy material, graded as mild, moderate, and severe [5].

Until now, tissue harvesting by scalpel biopsy and subsequent histological examination have been the gold standard for diagnosing premalignant and malignant oral diseases. Oral biopsy is invasive and involves both psychological implications for the patient and technical difficulties for the health practitioner. When lesions are

R. Mehrotra (✉)
Institute of Cytology and Preventive Oncology (ICPO), I-7, Sector - 39, Noida - 201301, Uttar Pradesh, India
e-mail: rm8509@gmail.com

R. Mehrotra (ed.), *Oral Cytology: A Concise Guide*, DOI 10.1007/978-1-4614-5221-8_1,

extensive, the most representative areas must be selected to avoid diagnostic errors. A high inter- and intra-observer variability of histological diagnoses for dysplasia is well documented and has been described by several authors [6, 7]. As highlighted in a study of 200 patients with oral leukoplakia, when two scalpel biopsies are performed at different times by different examiners, the agreement rate between them is only 56% [8]. The morphology of low grade dysplasia is significantly variable and a reproducible diagnosis is difficult. For high-grade dysplastic lesions, incisional biopsies of suspicious lesions, which have a limited reproducibility within the whole lesion, may result in a more or less aggressive surgical and/or radio-chemotherapeutic approach [9].

Identifying additional diagnostic tools would be welcome to improve analysis of any suspicious lesion. The oral cytology technique is simple, nonaggressive, relatively painless, and tolerated well by patients [10]. It can also be used for diagnosis and identification of recurrent potentially malignant and malignant lesions [11].

The basic requirements for a useful diagnostic technique include the following: ease to use, minimal patient discomfort, and collection of sufficient cells. Ideally, a diagnostic procedure should be neither time-consuming nor complicated and, in addition to high sensitivity, should have the potential for automation. Cytology meets all of these requirements, particularly when it is supplemented by a variety of novel adjunctive aids.

This book is an attempt to concisely bring to the reader a state of the art update on this, rather exotic, but increasingly important diagnostic modality.

References

1. American Cancer Society. Cancer facts & figures 2012. 2012. http://www.cancer.org/Cancer/OralCavityandOropharyngealCancer/DetailedGuide/oral-cavity-and-oropharyngeal-cancer-key-statistics. Accessed 1 Mar 2012.
2. Mehrotra R, Pandya S, Chaudhary AK, Kumar M, Singh M. Prevalence of oral premalignant and malignant lesions at a tertiary level hospital in Allahabad, India. Asian Pac J Cancer Prev. 2008;9:263–6.
3. Thomson PJ, Hamadah O. Cancerisation within the oral cavity: the use of 'field mapping biopsies' in clinical management. Oral Oncol. 2007;43:20–6.
4. Johnson NW. Orofacial neoplasms: global epidemiology, risk factors and recommendations for research. Int Dent J. 1991;41:365–75.
5. Pindborg JJ, Reichart PA, Smith CJ, Van Der Waal I. Histological typing of cancer and precancer of the oral mucosa. World Health Organisation. Berlin: Springer-Verlag; 1997. p. 21–314.
6. Warnakulasuriya S, Reibel J, Bouquot D, Dabelsteen E. Oral epithelial dysplasia classification systems: predictive value, utility, weaknesses and scope for improvement. J Oral Pathol Med. 2008;37:127–33.
7. Kujan O, Khattab A, Oliver RJ, Roberts SA, Thakker N, Sloan P. Why oral histopathology suffers inter-observer variability on grading oral epithelial dysplasia: an attempt to understand the sources of variation. Oral Oncol. 2007;43:224–31.
8. Lee JJ, Hung HC, Cheng SJ, et al. Factors associated with underdiagnosis from incisional biopsy of oral leukoplakic lesions. Oral Surg Oral Med Oral Pathol Oral Radiol Endod. 2007;104:217–25.

9. Holmstrup P, Vedtofte P, Reibel J, Stoltze K. Oral premalignant lesions: is a biopsy reliable? J Oral Pathol Med. 2007;36:262–6.
10. Driemel O, Kunkel M, Hullmann M, et al. Diagnosis of oral squamous cell carcinoma and its precursor lesions. J German Soc Derm. 2007;5:1095–100.
11. Moralis A, Kunkel M, Reichert TE, Kosmehl H, Driemel O. Identification of a recurrent oral squamous cell carcinoma by brush cytology. Mund Kiefer Gesichtschir. 2007;11:355–8.

Chapter 2
Historical Development of Oral Cytology

Vishal Dhingra and Ravi Mehrotra

Introduction

The seminal work by Papanicolaou and Traut in studying the cells from precancerous and cancerous lesions of the cervical mucosa paved the way for oral cytology. Their work proved an effective tool for screening gynecologic malignant disease [1]. Initially, the use of oral cytology was limited to comparative studies of oral and cervical cytology, describing cytomorphological changes depending on the menstrual cycle. Interestingly, buccal smears also have been reported to show marked cyclic fluctuation in keratinization during the normal menstrual cycle [2–4].

In the second half of the nineteenth century, the morphology of malignant cells in sputum was first described from an oropharyngeal carcinoma [5]. This was followed by work of Morrison et al. in which they used Papanicolaou staining to diagnose nasopharyngeal carcinomas [6]. But it was Montgomery and von Haam who were the first to examine the usefulness of cytology in the oral cavity [7]. Some further studies showed the application of oral cytology by animal experiments [8, 9]. Oral cytology has been used effectively as a research tool for the evaluation of experimentally induced carcinomas in hamster cheek pouches and in healing of gingivectomy wounds [10]. Much later, Sandler, through his series of reports on Veterans Administration studies of oral cytology, focused attention on the potential of the technique as an aid to early detection of oral cancer [11]. These landmarks in the development of oral exfoliative cytology are listed in Table 2.1.

V. Dhingra (✉)
Department of Pathology, Moti Lal Nehru Medical College,
Lowther Road, Allahabad, Uttar Pradesh 211002, India
e-mail: vishaldhingra9@yahoo.com

R. Mehrotra
Institute of Cytology and Preventive Oncology (ICPO), I-7, Sector - 39, Noida - 201301,
Uttar Pradesh, India
e-mail: rm8509@gmail.com

R. Mehrotra (ed.), *Oral Cytology: A Concise Guide*, DOI 10.1007/978-1-4614-5221-8_2,

Table 2.1 Landmarks in the development of oral exfoliative cytology

Year of publication	Author	Subject of publication
1860	Beale [5]	Cytological examination of sputum in a case of pharyngeal carcinoma
1940	Weinmann [12]	Cytological examination of oral cellular keratinisation
1941	Ziskin et al. [13]	Effects of the menstrual cycle on oral cellular morphology
1942	Papanicolaou [14]	Introduction of a staining procedure for cytological smears
1943	Papanicolaou and Traut [3]	Cytological diagnosis of uterine cancer
1949	Morrison et al. [6]	Cytological diagnosis of nasopharyngeal malignancies

Modified from J Oral Pathol Med (2009) 38: 161–166 R. Mehrotra et al.

Cytology Techniques and Their Modifications

Over a period of time, as the field of oral cytology started to grow, many investigators including Montgomery and von Haam experienced the limitations of oral cytology and therefore felt the need for improvements. They devised numerous modifications which were intended to procure larger amount of cells, to sample a large cellular area and also to improve the quality of cell staining. However these modifications were not put to widespread use. Special stains have been advocated, either to define the best area for cell collection in a diffuse lesion or to enhance the definition of malignant cells for the examining pathologist. Some of these have been listed in Table 2.2. In order to reach the cells of the basal and parabasal layers, the atypical keratotic cell layers need to be removed. It is for this very purpose, the use of a metal spatula or a sharp spoon was recommended by some authors [20, 21].

Besides these techniques, numerous supportive analytical methods for light microscopy were used. Possible utilization of fluorescence microscopy and phase contrast microscopy was investigated. Fluorescent DNA-specific dyes like Acridine Orange were used to measure the cellular DNA content [22]. Analysis of nucleolar size and diameter, as additional parameters for malignancy, was carried out with the help of image cytometry [23]. Besides the classical applications of the oral cytological studies, detection of Epstein–Barr virus in oral lesions of hairy leukoplakia has also been done, thereby widening its possibilities [24].

Oral Cytology in Cancer Detection

Oral cytology appeared to be a promising diagnostic tool as it was thought to have potential for early detection of malignant lesions. The issue of whether oral cytology could be applicable for mass population screening is somewhat unsettled,

Table 2.2 Methodical modifications of oral exfoliative cytology

Year of publication	Author	Modification in material and methods
1951	Gladstone [15]	Improved quantities of obtained cells by use of a "sponge biopsy"
1952	Schneider [16]	Modifications of staining
1960	Cawson [17]	Modifications of staining
1963	King [18]	Use of frosted glass slides
1963	Staats and Goldsby [19]	Comparison of wooden and metal spatula. Recommendation of the metal spatula
1964	Sandler [20]	Removal of keratotic layers with a sharp curette
1981	Dumbach et al. [21]	Smear curettage'. Inclusion of deeper cell layers by use of a curette

Modified from J Oral Pathol Med (2009) 38: 161–166 R. Mehrotra et al.

although the majority opinion seems to be that it was not practical at that time. Thus, investigators came up with numerous modifications in the techniques, some of which have been described above. These modifications did increase the sensitivity of cytology. However the main advantage of cytology was lost as compared with surgical biopsy as these kinds of scrapings were more invasive.

At the same time, oral cytology could not prove to be an effective tool for detecting early neoplastic lesion of the oral cavity in the way cervical cytology did. The reasons for this were manifold. First, oral topography and the size of the oral cavity made it virtually an impossible task to examine the complete mucosal surface. Thus, only the region which had visible lesions could be cytologically examined. It cannot be overemphasized that an adequate sample is essential if morphological evaluation of the collected cells is to yield representative findings. Even for histopathological examination, if a carcinoma covers a large area, it is important to carefully select the most appropriate site of the scalpel biopsy [25].

Secondly, a definite transformation zone as on the cervical mucosa, where malignant cells reach the epithelial surface in early tumor stages, does not exist in oral cancer [26]. Therefore, it was only possible to obtain malignant cells by conventional smears, if the carcinoma was fairly advanced or ulcerated [20]. Thus none of the existing minimally invasive techniques were able to sample deeper layers of the oral cavity—access to which was necessary to make oral cytology an effective preventive tool for oral cancers.

Conventional oral brush cytology has sensitivity ranging between 79% and 97% and specificity between 95.1% and 99.5%. Though there is an increase in the accuracy but this have not significantly increased compared with conventional exfoliative cytology. Thus, the need to improve analytics, which utilize technology like image analysis and automated machines, remains a challenge for the investigators.

Oral Brush

The introduction of the oral brush is a significant landmark in the history of oral cytology. Use of a brush for cervical cytology demonstrated better cell spreading on objective slides as well as an improvement in quality and validity of smears compared with smears obtained by using a wooden spatula [27]. But it is the ability of the oral brush to sample deeper mucosal layers, the site for squamous intra-epithelial lesions (SIL), with minimal invasion that is the principal basis for its success in oral cytology. [28]. It is a more convenient instrument, for the examiner, than the wooden tongue depressor, when dealing with oral lesions [26]. Moreover, this technique is a chair-side, easy to perform, painless test that can be used to evaluate any suspicious lesion, including common small white and red oral lesions, to rule out dysplasia.

A multicenter study emphasized the importance of brush biopsy with automated imaging in which clinically benign-appearing mucosal lesions were sampled using this technique and nearly 5% were later confirmed by using scalpel biopsy to represent dysplastic epithelial changes or invasive cancer [29]. Many other authors demonstrated that brush cytology could uncover similar lesions that were not clinically suspicious of carcinoma or pre-invasive disease [30]. Interestingly, a case report published a few years back emphasized the value of brush cytology in the follow-up of oral lesions which covered a large area [31]. In another report, Gupta et al. combined conventional oral brush cytology with the application of toluidine blue to localize the right site for brushing in suspected mucosal areas [32]. Mehrotra et al., in his study recently confirmed the utility of automated analysis in minimally suspicious (Class II) lesions [33].

Conclusions

Oral cytology has come a long way from its primitive Papanicolaou days. It has made major strides in its eventful development. The oral health professionals along with multidisciplinary scientific investigators have played a pivotal role in discovering optimal methods that would allow early diagnosis of oral cancer. Early detection should lead to less damage from cancer therapy and better prognosis. Surgical excision followed by a histopathological diagnosis, however, remains the widely accepted benchmark for the present. There are a number of recently introduced novel techniques that help in the diagnosis of oral malignancy. The future of these newer techniques appears extremely promising and should, hopefully, change the paradigm of oral cancer diagnostics.

References

1. Papanicolaou GN, Traut HF. Diagnosis of cancer by vaginal smears. New York: The Commonwealth Fund; 1943.
2. Papanicolaou GN. Atlas of exfoliative cytology. Cambridge: Harvard University Press; 1954.
3. Papanicolaou GN, Traut HF. Diagnosis of uterine cancer by the vaginal smear. New York: The Commonwealth Fund; 1943. p. S1–47.
4. Papanicolaou GN. A survey of the actualities and potentialities of exfoliative cytology in cancer diagnosis. Ann Intern Med. 1949;31:661–74.
5. Beale LS. Examination of sputum from case of cancer of the pharynx and adjacent parts. Arch Med. 1860;2:44–6.
6. Morrison LF, Hopp ES, Wu R. Diagnosis of malignancy of the nasopharynx. Cytological studies by the smear technique. Ann Otol Rhinol Laryngol. 1949;58:18–32.
7. Montgomery PW, von Haam E. A study of the exfoliative cytology in patients with carcinoma of the oral mucosa. J Dent Res. 1951;30:308–13.
8. Camilleri GE, Smith CJ. Exfoliative cytology in experimental oral carcinogenesis. Acta Cytol. 1964;8:85–90.
9. Hanks CT, Chaudhry AP, Neiders ME. Reliability of exfoliative cytology in induced carcinoma in hamster's pouch. Acta Cytol. 1969;13:94–8.
10. Stahl SS. Exfoliative cytology in an experimentally induced carcinoma of the hamster cheek pouch. Acta Cytol. 1963;7:262–7.
11. Sandler HC, Stahl SS. Exfoliative cytology as a diagnostic aid in the detection of oral neoplasms. J Oral Surg. 1958;16:414–8.
12. Weinmann J. The keratinization of the human oral mucosa. J Dent Res. 1940;19:57.
13. Ziskin DE, Kamen P, Kitley I. Epithelial smears from oral mucosa. J Dent Res. 1941;20:386–7.
14. Papanicolaou GN. A new procedure for staining vaginal smears. Science. 1942;95:438–9.
15. Gladstone SA. Sponge biopsy in the diagnosis of the cancer in the mouth. J Oral Surg. 1951;9:104–9.
16. Schneider G. Krebserkennung und zytodiagnostik. Dtsch Zahnarztl Z. 1952;7:1127–43.
17. Cawson RA. The cytological diagnosis of oral cancer. Br Dent J. 1960;19:294–8.
18. King OH. Intraoral exfoliative cytology technics. Acta Cytol. 1963;7:327–9.
19. Staats OJ, Goldsby JW. Graphic comparison of intra oral exfoliative cytology technics. Acta Cytol. 1963;7:107–10.
20. Sandler HC. The cytologic diagnosis of tumors of the oral cavity. Acta Cytol. 1964;8:114–20.
21. Dumbach J, Sitzmann F, Pesch HJ. Diagnostisches Vorgehen bei Verdacht auf Malignom der Mundho¨ hle unter besonderer Beru¨ cksichtigung der Exfoliativ-Zytologie. Dtsch Zahnarztl Z. 1981;36:697–700.
22. Caulder SL. Fluorescence microscopy utilizing acridine orange in oral cytodiagnosis. Oral Surg. 1967;23:343–50.
23. Abdel-Salam M, Mayall BH, Hansen LS, Chew KL, Greenspan JS. Nuclear DNA analysis of oral hyperplasia and dysplasia using image cytometry. J Oral Pathol. 1987;16:431–5.
24. Walling DM, Flaitz CM, Adler-Storthz K, Nichols CM. A non-invasive technique for studying oral epithelial Epstein–Barr virus infection and disease. Oral Oncol. 2003;39:436–44.
25. Mehrotra R, Gupta A, Singh M, Ibrahim R. Application of cytology and molecular biology in diagnosing premalignant or malignant oral lesions. Mol Cancer. 2006;5:1–11.
26. Ogden GR, Cowpe JG, Green M. Cytobrush and wooden spatula for oral exfoliative cytology. A comparison. Acta Cytol. 1992;36:706–10.
27. Murata PJ, Johnson RA, McNicoll KE. Controlled evaluation of implementing the cytobrush technique to improve Papanicolaou smear quality. Obstet Gynecol. 1990;75:690–5.
28. Boon ME, Alons-van Kordelaar JJM, Rietveld-Scheffers PEM. Consequences of the introduction of combined spatula and cytobrush sampling for cervical cytology improvements in smear quality and detection rates. Acta Cytol. 1986; 30: 264–70.

29. Ahmed HG, Idris AM, Ibrahim SO. Study of oral epithelial atypia among Sudanese tobacco users by exfoliative cytology. Anticancer Res. 2003;23:1943–9.
30. Mehrotra R, Singh MK, Pandya S, Singh M. The use of an oral brush biopsy without computer-assisted analysis in the evaluation of oral lesions: a study of 94 patients. Oral Surg Oral Med Oral Pathol Oral Radiol Endod. 2008;106:246–53.
31. Moralis A, Kunkel M, Reichert TE, Kosmehl H, Driemel O. Identifikation eines rezidivierenden, oralen Plattenepithelkarzinoms mittels Bu¨ rstenzytologie. Mund Kiefer Gesichtschir. 2007;11:355–8.
32. Gupta A, Singh M, Ibrahim R, Mehrotra R. Utility of toluidine blue and oral brush biopsy in oral precancerous lesions and squamous cell carcinoma. Acta Cytol. 2007;51:788–94.
33. Mehrotra R, Mishra S, Singh M, Singh M. The efficacy of oral brush biopsy with computer-assisted analysis in identifying precancerous and cancerous lesions. Head Neck Oncol. 2011;3:39.

Chapter 3
Oral Cytology Techniques

Kachnar Varma, Jos Hille, Amir Afrogheh, and Ravi Mehrotra

Examination of the oral cavity has traditionally been the preferred approach for detection of oral mucosal abnormalities. It is a noninvasive technique that can be performed quickly by a multitude of healthcare professionals without any additional expense to the patient.

The evidence regarding visual examination as an effective screening technique, however, remains controversial [1]. A randomized controlled trial with nearly 130,000 participants performed by the Kerala group in India demonstrated improved survival rates of up to 9 years only among men with high-risk habits (tobacco use) [2]. Although there was no increase in survival for the overall population, this study was the first to clearly support the efficacy of an oral cancer screening program in a high-risk subgroup. However, experts conclude that, presently, there is insufficient evidence to support or refute the use of oral examination, by itself, as an effective screening test.

Supravital Staining

Toluidine blue (TB) is an acidophilic dye designed to stain acidic cellular components, such as DNA and RNA. Its use in the detection of precancerous/cancerous tissue is based on the fact that dysplastic tissue contains quantitatively more DNA

K. Varma (✉)
Department of Pathology, Moti Lal Nehru Medical College,
412/4, MLN Medical College Campus, Allahabad, Uttar Pradesh, India
e-mail: varmakachnar@yahoo.co.in

J. Hille • A. Afrogheh
TBH Laboratories, Oral & Maxillofacial Pathology, University of the Western Cape,
National Health Laboratory Service, Cape Town, South Africa

R. Mehrotra
Institute of Cytology and Preventive Oncology (ICPO), I-7, Sector - 39, Noida - 201301,
Uttar Pradesh, India
e-mail: rm8509@gmail.com

R. Mehrotra (ed.), *Oral Cytology: A Concise Guide*, DOI 10.1007/978-1-4614-5221-8_3,

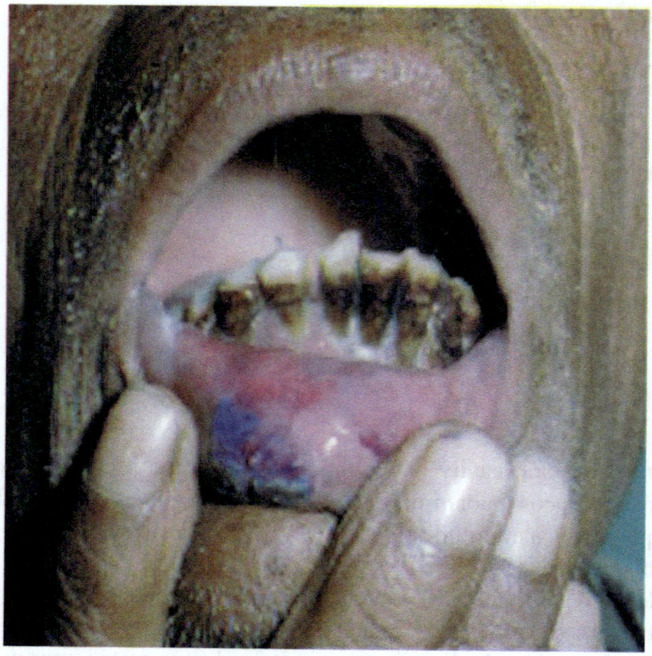

Fig. 3.1 Clinical picture of a patient with dysplasia of lower lip showing positive toluidine blue staining (Courtesy: Mehrotra et al [23].)

and RNA than non-dysplastic tissue. To perform the staining, the mucosal surface is wiped with 1% acetic acid solution as a mucolytic agent followed by the application of 1% to 2% Toluidine blue solution and the mucosa is blotted dry. The clinician then examines the oral mucosa for areas of increased cellular staining [3] as shown in Fig. 3.1. In the evaluation of a potentially malignant oral lesion, TB staining may provide better demarcation of lesion margins, guide biopsy site selection, and is thought to be valuable in identification and visualization of lesions in high-risk patients. Though useful as an adjunct to clinical examination, the specificity of TB staining is limited as cells undergoing inflammatory changes and benign hyperplasia may also retain dye leading to false-positive results. Overall, the sensitivity of TB staining ranges from 0.78 to 1.00 and the specificity from 0.31 to 1.00. Although 100% of cancers may stain, most studies show that only 50% or less of dysplasias are detected by this technique [4]. Similarly, Lugol's iodine has also been sucessfuly used for identifying clinically suspicious and minimally suspicious mucosal lesions (Fig. 3.2).

Exfoliative Cytology in Oral Lesions

A significant proportion of oral squamous cell carcinomas (OSCC) develop from pre-malignant lesions. Surgical biopsy remains the gold standard for diagnosis and identification of pre-malignant and malignant oral lesions, but it has many

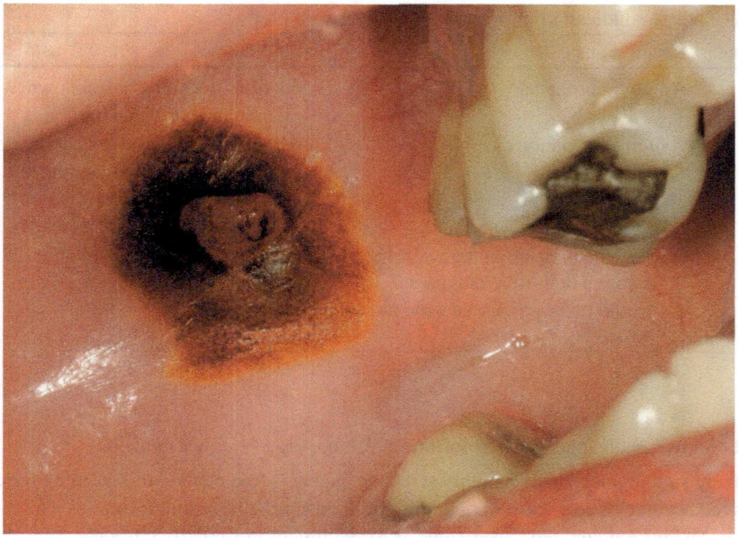

Fig. 3.2 Minimally suspicious (clinical Class II) oral mucosal lesion in the buccal mucosa stained with Lugol's iodine

disadvantages. It is an invasive procedure with technical limitations for professionals and psychological implications for most patients. Especially, it presents a problem when the lesions are large, as it is important to select the most appropriate site of biopsy in these cases [5]. On the other hand, exfoliative cytology is a simple, semi-invasive technique based on the concept that malignant cells adhere weakly to each other and thus are easier to harvest by scraping or brushing a suspicious tissue surface in a relatively atraumatic way. It enables the operator to collect a rich concentration of cells over a much wider area in comparison to surgical biopsy, so a small focus of malignancy is not easily missed. This technique may be employed usefully in combination with histology and is generally well tolerated by the patient [6]. The use of this methodology underlines the importance of discovering and developing new diagnostic techniques, improving the existing ones and discovering new adjuvant molecular targets for oral non-neoplastic and neoplastic diseases [7]. Indications for oral exfoliative cytology and biopsy are summarized in Table 3.1.

Advantages of Oral Exfoliative Cytology Over Biopsy (Table 3.2)

Exfoliative cytology is a useful and simple diagnostic procedure. It may be of value in noncompliant patients who is unlikely to come back for a follow-up examination or accept an immediate referral to the oral surgeon [8], and in medically compromised patients who would be exposed to unnecessary surgical risks. Advantages of exfoliative cytology over surgical biopsy, in summary, are that it is simple, semi-invasive, relatively painless, inexpensive, causes minimal patient discomfort, and

Table 3.1 Showing indication of punch biopsy and brush biopsy

Indication	Punch biopsy	Brush biopsy
1.	An obvious cancer	Evaluation of lesions of unknown significance or behavior
2.	A highly suspicious lesion	Larger surface mucosal lesions, which have been duly noted and have remained under observation only and should be analyzed on a periodic basis
3.	A lesion in a person at high risk for whom a definitive diagnosis would be necessary as soon as possible	Evaluation of lesions of unknown significance or behavior

Table 3.2 Showing advantages highly of oral brush biopsy over other methods

- Relatively simple, inexpensive, highly sensitive, and risk-free method of screening for cancer
- Improved accuracy due to ease in obtaining full transepithelial cellular samples
- Exposes lesions not clinically suspicious of carcinoma or pre-invasive disease
- Cytobrush is more convenient to clinician than the wooden tongue depressor during oral exfoliative cytology
- Provides a more even distribution of epithelial cells on a glass slide than the wooden/tongue depressor
- Cellular samples obtained by cytobrush can be used for cytomorphometry, DNA cytometry, and immunocytochemical analysis

collects sufficient cells for diagnostic purposes. It also facilitates prompt therapy without resorting to more time-consuming and expensive procedures, and it is useful in the selection of a representative area to be biopsied, if indicated [5, 6].

Collecting Instruments in Oral Exfoliative Cytology

Wooden/Metallic Spatula

Wooden tongue depressor, metal spatula, and cotton-tipped applicator (Fig. 3.3) were amongst the most commonly used instruments for oral exfoliative cytology (Table 3.3). However, these instruments were associated with some disadvantages. They may cause pain and tenderness when they are scraped or rolled over sensitive oral mucosa, and they are awkward to use in selected intraoral locations such as the mandibular, lingual and gingival regions because of their inflexible and long handles. Furthermore, the quality and quantity of epithelial cells collected with these instruments can vary markedly. Epithelial cells collected with the wooden tongue depressor and metal spatula often exhibit significant nuclear and cytoplasmic

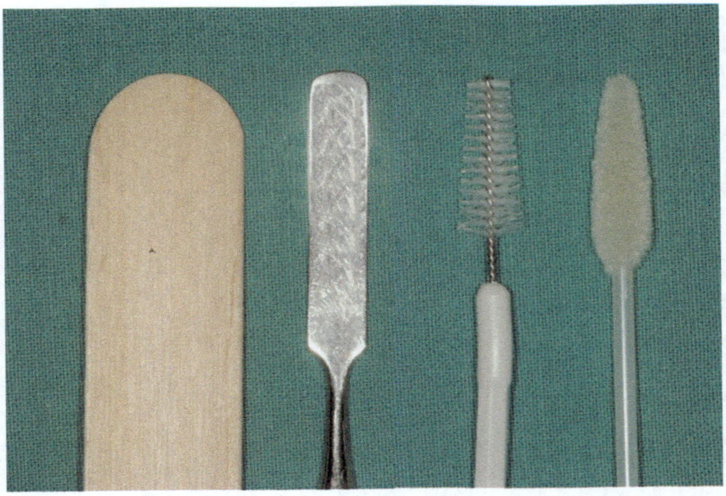

Fig. 3.3 Panel of exfoliative cytology collection devices (wooden tongue depressor, metal spatula, cervical brush, and flocked swab)

Table 3.3 Showing the sensitivity and specificity of different collecting devices for oral cytology

Collecting device	Sensitivity (%)	Specificity (%)
Cotton-tipped applicator/tongue depressor/ wooden spatula	86.5–97.5	88.9–100
Metal spatula	76.9–100	100
Curette	87–100	99.0
Conventional oral brush cytology	76.8–94.6	93.3–100

distortion [9]. This finding is related to the fact that these instruments tend to cluster the cells in thick aggregates. On the other hand, few epithelial cells are collected with the cotton-tipped applicator, possibly because of its nonadhesive surface and many cells being enmeshed in the cotton are not transferred to the slides. Wooden spatulas do not easily penetrate the often tougher keratotic surface layers, on the other hand, metal spatulas can be somewhat more invasive. The wooden spatula in particular lacks adequate flexibility in collecting diagnostic cells from areas of the oral cavity which are difficult to reach, such as the ventral surface of the tongue. The transfer of the amount of harvested cells from either a wooden to a glass slide is less than satisfactory; the porous and absorptive nature of the wooden spatula prevents adequate transfer of cellular material from the spatula to the glass slide producing paucicellular and nonrepresentative smears with clumping of the cells. Moreover a fair amount of mechanical damage to the cells can occur resulting from the friction of the rigid spatula surfaces with the glass during the transfer, causing problems in interpretation.

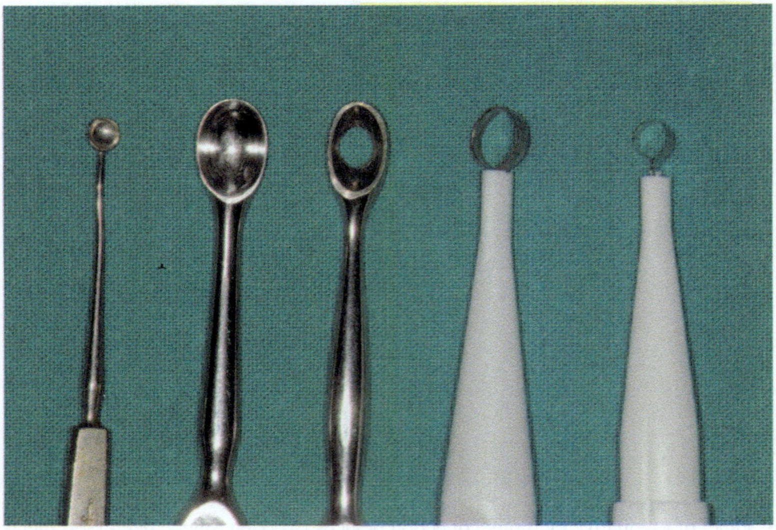

Fig. 3.4 Panel depicting different types of curettes

Disposable Dermatological Curette in Oral Cytology

Navone et al. used a disposable dermatological curette to sample potentially malignant lesions of the oral mucosa (Fig. 3.4). Although the invasive nature of this instrument results in adequate sampling of thick hyperkeratotic/leukoplakic lesions, its effectiveness over the more commonly used Cytobrush is yet to be proven. The dermatological curette with its rounded metallic tip geometry may cause significant patient discomfort [10].

Oral Cytobrush

Early investigators acknowledged the major limitations of oral exfoliative cytology and strove to improve the quality of the smears and the sampling procedure by modifying the collecting instruments, in an attempt to decrease the number of false negative results. Following the relatively high sensitivity of the cytobrush in diagnosing dysplastic lesions of the uterine cervix, the introduction of the softer straight endocervical brushes substantially improved the harvesting capacity of oral epithelial cells as they cling far better to the numerous bristle endings (Fig. 3.5). The cytobrush was also found to be less inconvenient to the patients than the blades or spatulas. However some difficulty in using the cervical cytobrushes with respect to their size and shape has been experienced and the development of a cytobrush suitable for oral sites with optimal size and bristle geometry is recommended [11].

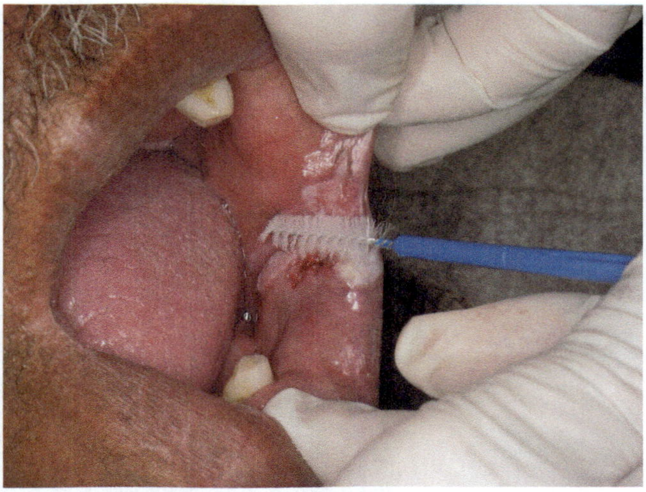

Fig. 3.5 Brushing of an oral lesion (Reprinted with permission, Afrogheh et al. [26])

Studies also suggest that there is limited accuracy of the conventional oral brush biopsy in the definitive diagnosis of potentially malignant and malignant oral lesions, particularly those less than 20 mm in diameter. The cervical cytobrush can also be used to make 2 parallel, identical smears (for different staining like Giemsa/Pap or even for immunocytochemistry) from the same cell sample by positioning the brush between two specimen slides using the thumb and index finger and rolling it under firm pressure from the label side towards the ends (Fig. 3.6). Conventional brush biopsy is most useful as an additional diagnostic tool for oral lesions, which are not highly suspicious for malignancy (clinical class II lesions) and therefore do not demand an immediate histological diagnosis [12].

Oral CDx-Patented Modification of Oral Brush

Computerized image analysis of brush biopsy samples (OralCDx Laboratories® Suffern, NY, USA) uses a computer program to perform morphologic and cytologic analysis of oral samples. The computerized analysis ranks cells based on abnormal morphology, which are then presented to a pathologist for further distinction and classification. The sensitivity of the OralCDx ranges from 0.71 to 1.00. This patented modification of the cervical brush into a circular configuration increases the yield of the deeper epithelial layers, since a higher rotational and more vigorous scraping pressure can be exerted on the surface of the lesion [13]. Figure 3.7 shows the Oral CDx cytobrush and collection kit. The improved accuracy is attributed to the ease in obtaining full transepithelial cellular samples and the evaluation of smears with an image analysis system that has been adapted specifically to detect

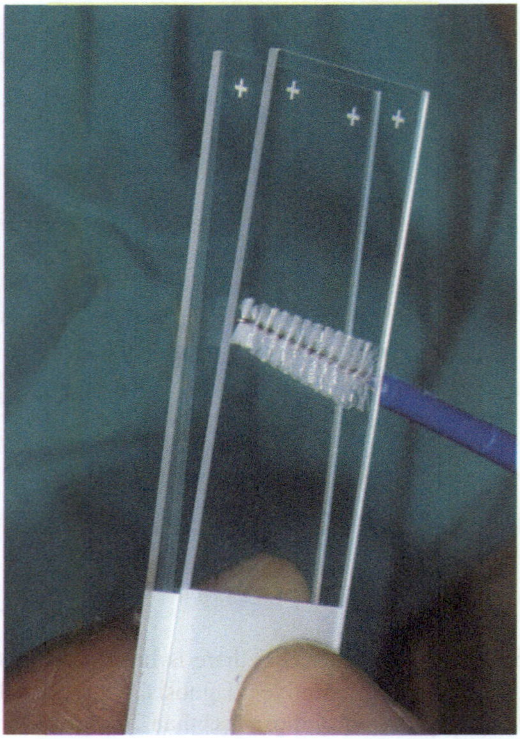

Fig. 3.6 Double slide-making technique with cervical brush positioned firmly between the glass slides

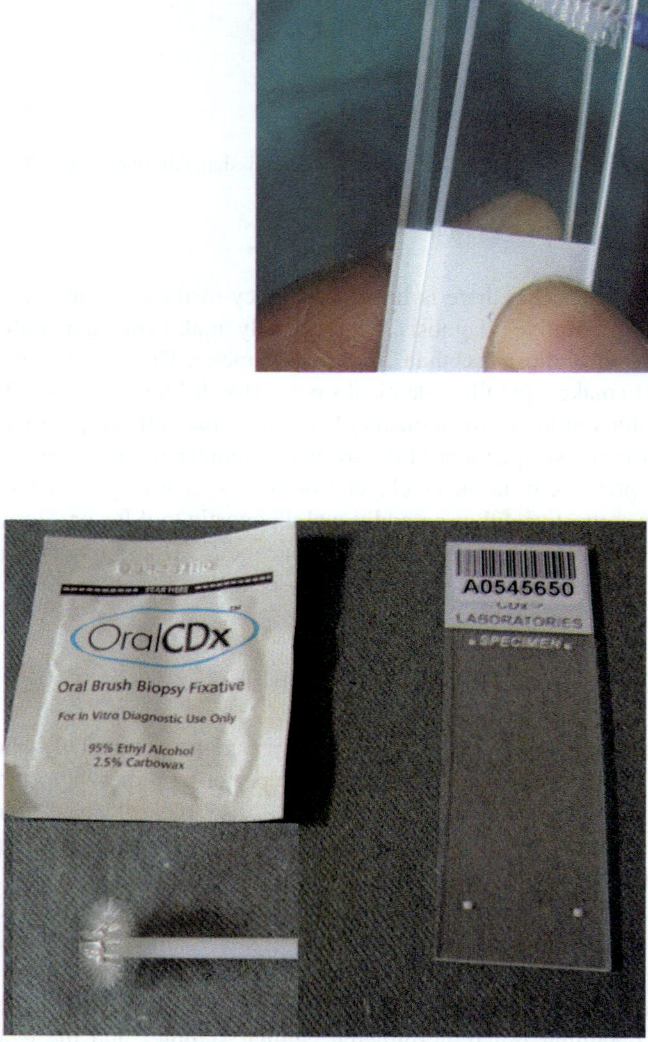

Fig. 3.7 The patented steel and plastic bristles of oral cytobrush of Oral CDx® kit

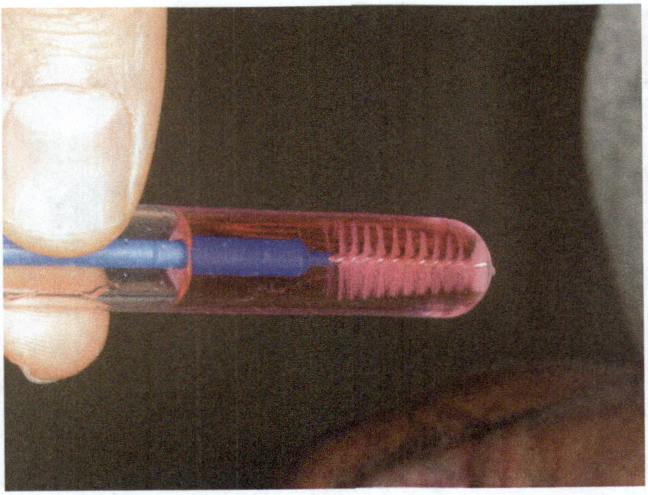

Fig. 3.8 Brush immersed and rinsed in LBC liquid (Reprinted with permission, Afrogheh et al. [26])

oral epithelial abnormalities. Full-thickness sampling (indicated by pinpoint bleeding during procedure is essential if cytomorphological evaluation of the collected cells is to yield representative findings. This has made it possible to penetrate a thick hyperkeratotic lesion, which otherwise prevents a thorough, full epithelial harvest, and to yield an adequate sample of the deeper and basal cell layers. This is of particular importance, since many dysplastic and invasive cells are first detected in the basal cell layer and the diagnostic cytomorphological features may be lost as the cells mature towards the surface and parakeratin/keratin are produced. It is well known that invasive oral carcinoma can occur in hyperplastic and hyperkeratotic precursor lesions [14].

Liquid-Based Cytology

Most recent advances in cytological procedures have led to the emergence of liquid-based cytology (LBC) in an attempt to improve the sensitivity of conventional cytological smears. The technique results in cellular preparations with reduced necrosis, blood contamination and inflammation. In liquid-based preparations, the collecting device is rinsed in a vial containing preservative fluid with even distribution, immediate fixation and significantly increased capture of the sampled cells, as seen in Fig. 3.8. There are currently two well established automated LBC methods. The Thin Prep (Cytyc Corporation, Boxborough, MA) obtained clearance from the Food and Drug Administration (FDA) in 1996, followed by the SurePath (BD TriPath,

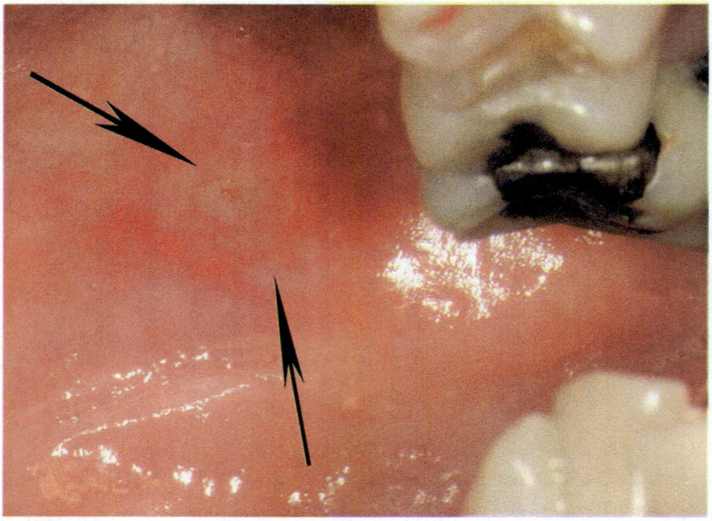

Fig. 3.9 This class II lesion in the buccal mucosa (in between arrows) showed high-grade atypia on liquid-based cytology brushings and invasive squamous carcinoma on biopsy

Burlington, NC) system, previously known as the AutoCyte Prep, in 1999 [15]. In the oral cavity, liquid based cytology is indicated in clinically suspicious (class I) and, more specifically, minimally suspicious (class II) lesions (Fig 3.9).

Oral Liquid Based Cytology

While a number of papers on cervical LBC have been published, there have been very few studies on oral LBC. In one of the first few comparative liquid based cytologic studies in the oral cavity and using a split-sample design, Hyama et al. reported a high diagnostic agreement between liquid-based preparations and conventional smears in oral lesions [16]. However, the thin-layer preparations demonstrated a statistically higher improvement in cell distribution (66%) and a substantial reduction in the presence of obscuring blood. Moreover, the number of inadequate specimens decreased and the cytomorphologic features were greatly enhanced with optimal visualization of viral cytopathic effects (e.g. HSV) and cytological abnormalities associated with squamous cell carcinoma [16].

In a study of normal oral mucosa using the Thin Prep LBC technique, Kujan et al. reported high quality specimens. Even distribution of cells, reduced clumping of epithelial cells and a marked reduction in the number of polymorphs, bacteria and mucus were noted. This led to ease of interpretation and significant reduction in screening time. Only 2 out of 150 specimens (1.3%) were considered inadequate [11].

In the one and only "high quality" (biopsy was used as gold standard for diagnostic comparison) LBC study from Italy, LBC was shown to have a better sensitivity (95.1%) and specificity (99%) than conventional cytology (85.7% sensitivity and 95.9% specificity) in the diagnosis of potentially malignant lesions of the oral mucosa, with fewer inadequate specimens, 8.8% in the LBC group versus 12.4% in the conventional cytology group [10]. On the other hand, the high unit cost of automated LBC techniques has led to the development of an alternative, manual, cost effective and competent cytopreparatory method based on cytocentrifugation, the Shandon PapSpin.

Cytocentrifugation

The technique utilizes the most common and readily available laboratory equipment, the Shandon Cytospin, while generating a cytologic sample of cells, easily interpreted using traditional and well-known cytomorphologic criteria [17].

In the first landmark comparative study using the new Shandon PapSpin LBC technique, Weynand et al. found no major differences in test performance between the new technique and conventional smears. However, the PapSpin produced excellent quality smears with a dramatic reduction in the "satisfactory but limited by…" specimens. An even distribution of cells was observed with fewer thick cellular aggregates and blood was not a feature in any of the PapSpin samples. The inflammatory cells were preserved but did not obscure the squamous elements. HPV testing was also possible using the PapSpin collection fluid [18].

Weynand and associates also reported a marked difference in the detection rate of fungal infections in favor of the PapSpin. They concluded that this technique's performance is equivalent to the FDA cleared automated LBC procedures but that the new technique eliminates the need for expensive equipments to prepare slides, making it a cost-effective alternative for automated LBC in cervical cancer screening. In a subsequent comparative study designed to optimize the new technique, Rosenthal et al. confirmed the earlier observations reported by Weynand et al. and mentioned that the new technique not only improves the screening time but effectively lowers the processing time [17]. With this technique, 48 PapSpin samples can be processed in 1 h, while 25 Thin Prep samples are processed in 1 h using the expensive T2000 equipment. It was also emphasized that PapSpin interpretation is not hampered since traditional cytomorphology is maintained and the background is preserved and dramatically improved.

Oral Brush Biopsy and Molecular Methods

It has recently been demonstrated that RNA can be extracted from exfoliated cells, and the use of RNA obtained by exfoliative cytology to determine susceptibility to cancer among healthy populations and detect early markers of carcinogenesis has

Table 3.4 Showing adjunctive techniques applied to brush biopsy specimen

- Quantitative cytomorphology
- Nuclear DNA content analysis
- Immunohistochemical tumor marker identification
- Molecular analysis
- Epigenetic alterations (promoter hypermethylation)
- Genomic instability and loss of heterozygosity (LOH)
- Microsatellite instability (MSI) and restriction fragment length polymorphism (RFLP)

therefore been proposed. Various adjunctive methods which can be applied with oral brush biopsy have been summarized in Table 3.4. Epigenetic alterations (promoter hypermethylation), genomic instability and loss of heterozygosity (LOH), microsatellite instability (MSI), and restriction fragment length polymorphism (RFLP) are other molecular markers that are being used [19].

Fine Needle Aspiration Biopsy in Oral Lesions

In the oral cavity, fine needle aspiration biopsy (FNAB) is indicated for biopsies of palpable nodules (deep mucosal abnormalities) not amenable to oral exfoliative cytology. Oral exfoliative cytology is best reserved for epithelial abnormalities (such as leukoplakia, erythroplakia and ulcerating squamous cell carcinoma). FNAB is widely used in organs of the head and neck regions, such as in the thyroid, lymph nodes, major salivary glands and other neoplasia, but rarely employed in the oral region [20].

The accessibility of most intra-oral nodules makes them ideal for fine-needle aspiration as part of pre-operative and post-operative (clinical follow-up) assessment. Reactive (e.g. fibroepithelial polyp, pyogenic granuloma, peripheral giant cell granuloma and calcifying fibrous epulis), cystic (e.g. gingival cyst of the adult, mucoceles) and neoplastic lesions are the most commonly encountered lesions.

The neoplastic lesions are primarily of salivary gland (e.g. pleomorphic adenoma) soft tissue (e.g. schwannomas, Kaposi's sarcoma), lymphoid (e.g. plasmablastic lymphoma) and odontogenic origin (e.g. peripheral variants of most odontogenic tumors). The technique is simple, quick and well tolerated by the patient. It is generally safe to perform and has a low risk of infection and tissue damage. Potential drawbacks include the largely unfounded, possibility of seeding of the tumor along the needle track or into surrounding tissues and hemorrhage. A great disadvantage is that the oral cavity provides limited space to perform the cutting movements required during the FNAB procedure. A more significant practical difficulty is the possibility that the technique may lead to traumatic artifacts in the excision specimen. These include intra-tumoral hemorrhage inflammation, fibrosis and squamous metaplasia, which may have a pseudoepitheliomatous appearance. Fine-needle aspiration biopsy is most

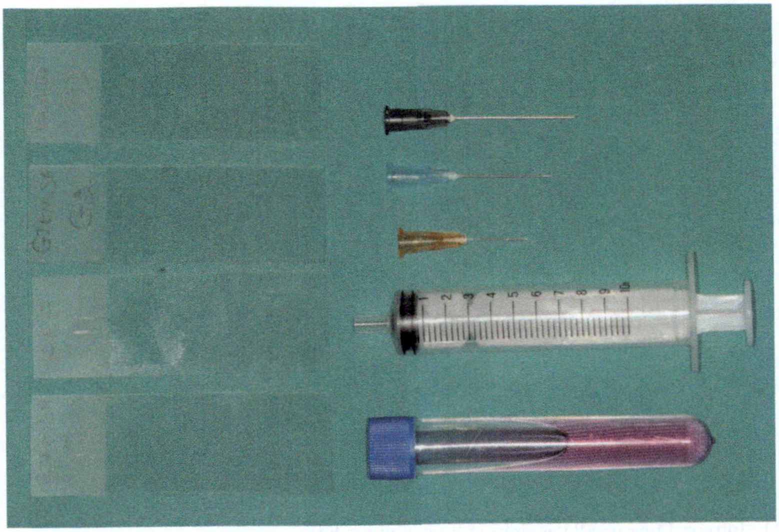

Fig. 3.10 Fine needle aspiration set

useful when the investigating clinician asks a series of questions rather than expecting an absolutely precise diagnosis. Such questions might include:

- Is the lesion reactive, cystic or neoplastic?
- If neoplastic, is it likely to be benign or malignant?
- Is it primary or metastatic?
- If cystic, could it be of salivary gland origin?

Using a series of these or similar questions can frequently prevent unnecessary or disproportionate surgery [21]. It is also important to understand some of the factors that can potentially compromise the interpretation of fine needle aspiration biopsies. It is critical that some of these limitations are explained to the patient before undertaking major surgical procedures on the basis of such a biopsy.

These limitations include the diverse nature and range of minor salivary gland tumors, the presence of cells such as myoepithelial cells in both benign and malignant tumors and the overlapping cytological features in minor salivary gland neoplasms (e.g. pseudocystic spaces in polymorphous low grade adenocarcinoma, adenoid cystic carcinoma and pleomorphic adenoma). All these potential problems can be exacerbated by sampling limitations. An example is sampling the pleomorphic adenoma component of carcinoma ex pleomorphic adenoma [22]. The most common diagnostic problem reported with FNAB of the oral cavity is insufficient amount of material collected for analysis [20]. In the oral cavity, the sensitivity of FNAB may vary from 80 to 100%; specificity varies from 80 to 100% and the accuracy varies from 60 to 100%. The false positive rate has been reported to vary from 0 to 3% and the false negative rate from 0 to 20% [23, 24].

The FNAB is usually performed with a 20 ml syringe and a 23 or 25 gauge needle (Fig. 3.10). Given the sensitive nature of the oral mucosal sites it may, at

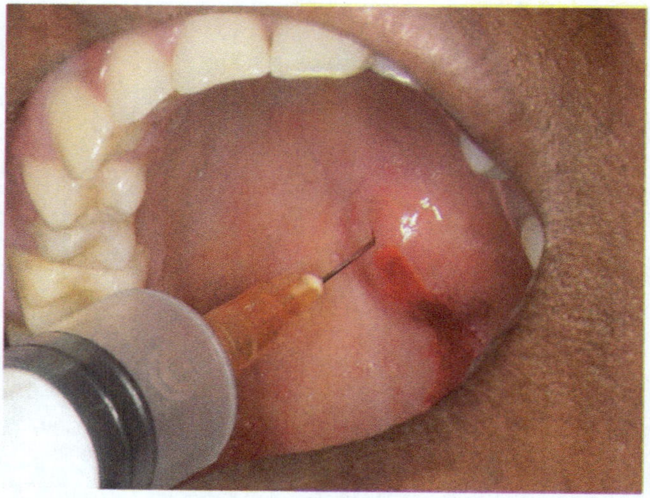

Fig. 3.11 Intraoral fine needle aspiration biopsy procedure

times, be advisable to apply a topical anesthetic (ideally 0.2% Xylotox/Lignocaine spray) prior to the procedure. After that, the needle is inserted into the lesion, and a vacuum is created and maintained, while the operator proceeds with the cutting movements at different angles throughout the lesion. Once sufficient material is seen in the hub of the needle, the pressure is released and the needle is withdrawn from the lesion (Fig. 3.11). The needle is then removed from the syringe, which is filled with air. The needle is repositioned back onto the syringe and placed near the surface of two glass slides, on which the collected material is deposited. One slide is immediately spray fixed (Pap) and the other air dried (for Giemsa or PAS, etc.). When aspirating cysts, the cystic content must be fully drawn and then aspirated again to obtain material from the capsule. Aspirates with large amount of blood content must be discarded to allow better interpretation of smears.

DNA Image Cytometry

In this method fluorescent DNA-specific dyes, such as acridine orange, are used to measure the cellular DNA content and has been discussed in detail in later chapters [25].

Thus, to conclude, a variety of methods of varying degrees of sophistication and requiring different levels of technical expertise have been used to obtain cytological material from the oral cavity. It is expected that over the next few years, simpler and more sensitive methodology will be in place, thus making the technique not only widely acceptable and standardized, but also available to the patients who really require low-cost sensitive diagnostic tests.

References

1. Peacock ZS, Pogrel A, Schmidt BL. Exploring the reasons for delay in treatment of oral cancer. J Am Dent Assoc. 2008;139:1346–52.
2. Sankaranarayanan R, Ramadas K, Thomas G, et al. Effect of screening on oral cancer mortality in Kerala, India: a cluster-randomised controlled trial. Lancet. 2005;365:1927–33.
3. Trullenque-Eriksson A, Muñoz-Corcuera M, Campo-Trapero J, Cano-Sánchez J, Bascones-Martínez A. Analysis of new diagnostic methods in suspicious lesions of the oral mucosa. Med Oral Patol Oral Cir Bucal. 2009;14:210–6.
4. Epstein JB, Sciubba J, Silverman Jr S, Sroussi HY. Utility of toluidine blue in oral premalignant lesions and squamous cell carcinoma: continuing research and implications for clinical practice. Head Neck. 2007;29:948–58.
5. Hopper C, Kalavrezos N. Oral cytology: the surgical perspective. Cytopathology. 2007;18:329–30.
6. Glennie HRR, Gilbert JG, Melcher DH, Linehan J, Wadsworth PV. The place of cytology in laryngeal diagnosis. Clin Otolaryngol. 1976;1:131–6.
7. Mehrotra R, Hullmann M, Smeets R, Reichert TE, Driemel O. Oral cytology revisited. J Oral Pathol Med. 2009;38:161–6.
8. Lingen MW, Kalmar JR, Karrison T, Speight PM. Critical evaluation of diagnostic aids for the detection of oral cancers. Oral Oncol. 2008;44:10–22.
9. Ogden GR, Cowpe JG, Green M. Cytobrush and wooden spatula for oral exfoliative cytology. A comparison. Acta Cytol. 1992;36:706–10.
10. Navone R, Burlo P, Pich A, Pentenero M, Broccoletti R, Marsico A, et al. The impact of liquid-based oral cytology on the diagnosis of oral squamous dysplasia and carcinoma. Cytopathology. 2007;18:356–60.
11. Kujan O, Desai M, Sargent A, Bailey A, Turner A, Sloan P. Potential applications of oral brush cytology with liquid-based technology: results from a cohort of normal oral mucosa. Oral Oncol. 2006;42:810–8.
12. Koch FP, Kunkel M, Biesterfeld S, Wagner W. Diagnostic efficiency of differentiating small cancerous and precancerous lesions using mucosal brush smearsof the oral cavity—a prospective and blinded study. Clin Oral Invest. 2011;15(5):763–9.
13. Sciubba JJ. Improving detection of precancerous and cancerous oral lesions. Computer assisted analysis of the oral brush biopsy. U.S. Collaborative OralCDx Study Group. J Am Dent Assoc. 2002;133:272–4.
14. Mehrotra R, Gupta A, Singh M, Ibrahim R. Application of cytology and molecular biology in diagnosing premalignant or malignant oral lesions. Mol Cancer. 2006;5:1–9.
15. Hutchinson ML, Isenstein LM, Goodman A, Hurley AA, Douglass KL, Mui KK, et al. Homogeneous sampling accounts for the increased diagnostic accuracy using the Thin Prep processor. Am J Clin Pathol. 1994;101:215–9.
16. Hayama FH, Motta AC, Silva AG, Migliari DA. Liquid-based preparations versus conventional cytology: specimen adequacy and diagnostic agreement in oral lesions. Med Oral Patol Oral Cir Bucal. 2005;10:115–22.
17. Rosenthal DL, Geddes S, Trimble CL, Carson KA, Alli PM. The PapSpin: a reasonable alternative to other, more expensive liquid-based papanicolaou tests. Cancer Cytopathol. 2006;108:137–42.
18. Weynand B, Berliere M, Haumont E, Massart F, Pourvoyeur A, Bernard P, et al. A new liquid-based cytology technique. Acta Cytol. 2003;47:149–53.
19. Reboiras-López MD, Pérez-Sayáns M, Somoza-Martín JM, Gayoso-Diz P, Barros-Angueira F, Gándara-Rey JM, García-García A. Comparison of the Cytobrush(®), dermatological curette and oral CDx(®) brush test as methods for obtaining samples of RNA for molecular analysis of oral cytology. Cytopathology. 2012;23(3):192–7.
20. Candido dos Santos AP, Sugaya NN, dos Santos Pinto Junior D, Lemos Junior CA. Fine needle aspiration biopsy in the oral cavity and head and neck region. Braz Oral Res. 2011;25: 186–91.

21. Ellis GL, Auclair PL. Comparison of fine-needle aspiration biopsy with intraoperative frozen section. AFIP atlas of tumour pathology: tumours of the salivary glands, 4th series. Washington DC: American Registry of Pathology; 2008. 32–4.
22. Eveson W. Salivary tumours. Periodontology. 2000;2011:150–9.
23. Saleh HA, Clayman L, Marsi H. Fine needle aspiration biopsy of intraoral and oropharyngeal mass lesions. Cytojournal. 2008;5:4.
24. Shah SB, Singer MI, Liberman E, Ljung BM. Transmucoal fine-needle aspiration diagnosis of intraoral and intrapharyngeal lesions. Laryngoscope. 1999;109:1232–7.
25. Bouquot JE, Farthing PM, Speight PM. The pathology of oral cancer and precancer revisited. Curr Diag Path. 2006;12:11–21.
26. Afogheh A, Wright CA, Sellars SL, Pelsar A, Wetter J, Schubert PT, Hille J. An evaluation of the Shandon PapSpin liquid based oral test utilizing a novel cytologic scoring system. Oral Surg Oral Med Oral Pathol Oral Radiol. 2012;113:799–807.

Chapter 4
Diagnosis of Infectious Diseases by Oral Cytology

Mamta Singh, Rahela Ibrahim, and Ravi Mehrotra

Introduction

The importance of cytology in the diagnosis of various infective diseases has gained by leaps and bounds in the last few decades. The diagnosis is made by examining the cytomorphological changes, accompanying inflammatory reaction, and at times, identification of causative organisms. Recently, the pattern of oral infection has changed due to overuse of antibiotics, dietary and addiction habits, poor hygiene, illiteracy, low socioeconomic, and poor immune status. This change in immune status may be seen in human immunodeficiency virus (HIV) infection, terminal stages of many bacterial or parasitic infections causing immune suppression or paralysis, chemotherapy after tissue transplantation, malignancies, steroid therapy, and radiation. This chapter reviews the cytomorphological approach to diagnose various bacterial, fungal, parasitic, and viral infections. Cytology of the oral smears prepared by scraping (cytobrush or spatula), fine needle aspiration, and other techniques directly identify infectious agents or can indirectly assess changes by cytopathic effects in epithelial cells and type of inflammatory reaction.

M. Singh (✉)
Department of Pathology, Moti Lal Nehru Medical College,
19A/23, CY Chintamani Road, Darbhanga Colony, Allahabad, Uttar Pradesh, India
e-mail: mrspath@gmail.com

R. Ibrahim
Department of Pathology, Moti Lal Nehru Medical College,
C-301, G.T.B.Nagar, Kareli, Allahabad, Uttar Pradesh, India
e-mail: rahela_biotech@sify.com

R. Mehrotra
Institute of Cytology and Preventive Oncology (ICPO), I-7, Sector - 39, Noida - 201301,
Uttar Pradesh, India
e-mail: rm8509@gmail.com

R. Mehrotra (ed.), *Oral Cytology: A Concise Guide*, DOI 10.1007/978-1-4614-5221-8_4,

Infective Oral Cytology

The oral epithelium renews itself rapidly (approximately in 10–15 days). This rate is exaggerated during inflammation or infection. Direct sampling from the lesion gives accurate results of screening for inflammatory, dysplastic, or malignant lesions. The appearance, proportion of epithelial cells, and accompanying cells depend on the anatomical site of collection of sample for oral cytology. Atypical changes in epithelial cells may be seen in ulceration and non-specific inflammation due to irritation. These changes may be such, that without variation in size of the cells; nuclei may be single or multiple and chromocenters may exhibit changes that may be confused with malignant lesions. Inflammation of the oral cavity may be acute or chronic and infective or noninfective in origin; and clinically presents as ulceration or erosion, which in turn, may be diffuse or localized; single or multiple. Due to inflammation, there is an increased rate of desquamation of epithelial cells, so much so, that superficial and intermediate epithelial cells may be partially or even totally replaced by the deeper parabasal squamous cells. Cytoplasm may be poorly preserved and show cytopathic effects in the form of granulation, vacuolization, perinuclear clearing, or halos. The background of inflammatory oral smears may be proteinaceous or hemorrhagic with the presence of polymorphonuclear leucocytes, eosinophils, mast cells, mono or multinuclear macrophages, lymphocytes, and plasma cells, depending on the type and cause of inflammation as well as the nutritional and immune status of individual.

Acute infections: In acute infections, normally fine needle aspiration cytology (FNAC) is not recommended, unless it is imperative. In pyogenic infections, frank pus is aspirated which may be mixed with blood in varying proportions; smears reveal pus cells and macrophages, in addition to changes in epithelial cells. Most of the times, the cytoplasm is poorly preserved and is eosinophilic, can also show degenerative changes like single or multiple vacuoles and eosinophilic granules. After death of the cell due to chemotaxis, polymorphs are seen attached to the cell—even covering and obscuring the degenerated cell completely. Since Giemsa is a supravital stain, often degenerated cells are not properly visualized, then Papanicolaou or Hematoxylin & Eosin stain is advised. Since cells desquamate very fast during inflammation, deeper cells like parabasal squamous cells show variation in size and shape. Often these cells have relatively large, occasionally multiple, oval, or round vesicular nuclei, usually of monotonous size with visible chromocenters and sometimes, a small nucleoli. Microorganisms like Streptococci, Staphylococci, Pneumococci, Klebsiella and other gram-negative bacilli, acid fast bacilli, fungi and other microorganisms may be seen in the smears—especially in untreated cases. For exotic microorganisms, special stains are accordingly used if required, and finally identified by culture and advanced ancillary techniques.

Chronic infections: After the acute phase of disease, it usually passes to a subacute phase, followed by the chronic phase of inflammation due to the infection. In nonspecific chronic infections, fewer epithelial cells are seen as compared to the acute phase, along with mononuclear cells—lymphocytes, macrophages with or

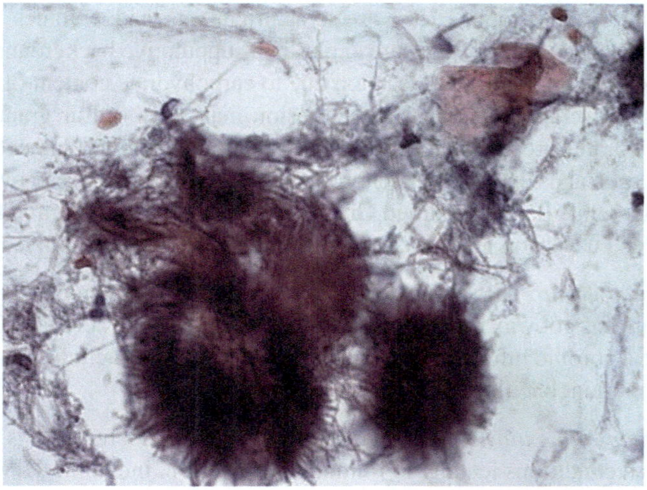

Fig. 4.1 Actinomyces colonies, epithelial squames, degenerated epithelial cells showing bare nuclei, inflammatory cells, and occasional red blood cells

without tingible bodies, plasma cells and, sometimes, occasional fibroblasts, or endothelial cells. Plenty of lymphocytes may be seen if aggressive scrape smears are made from tonsillar area, base of tongue or Waldeyer's ring.

Foreign body giant cells may be seen along with chronic inflammatory cells like—in cases of giant cell epulis. In rhinoscleroma, occasionally nasopharyngeal or pharyngeal smears show Mikulicz cells along with a chronic inflammatory reaction. They are identified morphologically as a macrophage, not as a plasma cell. The vacuoles observed in these cells are considered to be phagosomes containing bacterial mucopolysaccharides and swollen mitochondria [1]. If oral smears are contaminated with blood, sometimes, hemoparasites like microfilaria, *Plasmodium vivax*, *Plasmodium falciparum*, and other may be found as an accidental finding. There are few organisms which require special mention:

Bacterial Infections

Actinomycosis: Although the term actinomycosis seems to be a fungal infection, it is a subacute or chronic cervicofacial bacterial infection, caused by filamentous, branching, gram-positive anaerobic bacteria and is a normal saprophytic component of the oral flora—especially in the tonsillar crypts. *Actinomyces israelii*, *A. viscous*, and other species in synergism with Streptococci and Staphylococci cause infection [2]. There is very limited data on the role of FNAC in diagnosing these lesions [3]. The main reason for a missed cytodiagnosis in two thirds of the cases appeared to be observer error, thus it is suggested that when the aspiration smear from a mass is found to be an inflammatory exudate rich in neutrophils (Fig. 4.1), special efforts must be made to look for this microorganism [4].

In cytological preparations, it is seen as fragments and colonies of slender filamentous branches, usually, at acute angles in a suppurative background [5] along with a neutrophilic inflammatory reaction due to carbohydrate content of the organism. Aspirate or scrape material from the lesion may show sulfur granules which reveals a dark granular center and peripherally radiating numerous filamentous organisms in a necrotic and suppurative background [6]. They are easily seen by stains like Periodic Acid Schiff (PAS), modified Gram and Silver stains, if required fluorescent techniques can be used on granules, especially to identify the Actinomyces species.

Mycobacterium group: This group consists of many nonpathogenic and pathogenic organisms and has got wax in their cell wall which makes them acid fast. Pathogenic strains cause a chronic infection in various parts of the body-including the oral cavity. Some important bacilli are as follows:

Mycobacterium tuberculosis: Although the incidence of tuberculosis is increasing due to various conditions leading to immune suppression, including HIV infection, the incidence of oral lesions due to it are rare, being less than 1% of all tubercular lesions—mostly limited to the tonsils. Scrape or FNAC smears may show typical granulomatous findings—central caseation surrounded by multinucleated giant cells–Langhans giant cells, epithelioid cells lymphocytes, and plasma cells. Sometimes, only caseation and epithelioid cells are seen along with chronic inflammation, it is only rarely pus cells are found in necrotic background. Nearly 30% cases may be misdiagnosed as a chronic nonspecific inflammation. Bacilli are identified by acid fast stain. If it is negative, then repeat FNAC or various techniques like immunofluorescence [7], polymerase chain reaction (PCR) and culture can be used to confirm the diagnosis.

Mycobacterium leprae: It causes a chronic infectious disease also called Hansen's disease [8], which affects mainly the peripheral cooler parts of the body especially skin, testes, hands and feet, peripheral nerves, anterior chamber of the eye, upper airways up to the larynx including nasal cavity and hard palate. The clinical presentation depends on the immune status of the individual; in cases with good immunity it presents as tuberculoid leprosy and in cases of poor immunity it presents as lepromatous leprosy.

In *lepromatous leprosy*, when the lesion involves the nasal septum and hard palate, it presents as an ulcer and scrape smears show necrosis (caseous) along with either acute or chronic inflammatory reaction and lipid laden macrophages, (lepra cells) often filled with masses of acid fast bacilli (globi) [9], present freely in the smear.

In *tuberculoid leprosy*, smears may show chronic granulomatous lesions with or without bacilli and nonspecific chronic inflammatory lesions with bacilli. Low bacterial levels are seen in the mucosa, with or without ulceration in this group (tuberculoid and borderline patients) [10]. The bacterial count is low in tuberculoid as compared with lepromatous leprosy. Better results are seen by immuno or fluorescent stains and other ancillary techniques [11].

Mycoplasma: Mycoplasma are gram-negative coccobacilli that lack a cell wall. In immunocompromised patients, *M. orale* and *M. salivarium* may cause oral infections [12], presenting as mild to moderate inflammation, clinically present as sore

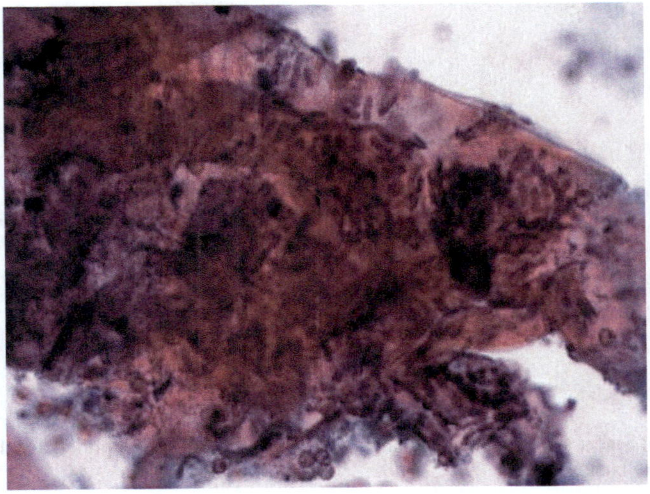

Fig. 4.2 Oral smear shows clumps of epithelial degenerated cells with Simonsiella infection

throat, the organism enters through cracks or abrasion in the skin. Infection causes local erythema and nodules at the site of inoculation, and can cause painful ulcers in the oral cavity.

The oropharyngeal mucosa, external nares, and conjunctival sacs are the preferred sampling sites, and oral smears show a nonspecific mixed inflammatory infiltrate by Giemsa stains. A definitive diagnosis is based on isolation and identification of the causative agent [13]. If required, the final diagnosis is made by serology [12] and other ancillary techniques.

Saprophytes and commensals: These are a group of organisms which are normally not pathogenic, but cause disease in immunocompromised patients. They include *Streptococcus sanguis*, *Streptococcus mutans*, *Propionibacterium acnes*, *Peptostreptococcus prevotii*, *Fusobacterium nucleatum*, *Prevotella intermedia*, *Saccharomyces cerevisiae*, *Peptostreptococcus micros*, *Vellonella*, *Streptococcus intermedius*, and *Streptococcus sanguis*, *Legionella* species and Simonsiella. (Fig. 4.2) Most of them can be recognized by culture; whilst others are non culturable.

Unculturable bacteria: *Bacteroides forsythus*, *Eubacterium*, *Porphyromonas*, *Gingivalis*, *Campylobacter rectus*, *Helicobacter pylori*, etc. They cause lesions in immunocompromised patients such as a rash or ulceration. Smears show mixed inflammatory reaction and the final diagnosis is made by employing various ancillary techniques.

Parasitic Infections

Leishmania: It is a chronic inflammatory disease of skin, mucous membranes or viscera caused by obligate intracellular, kinetoplastid protozoan parasites. Leishmania group of parasites is transmitted through the bite of infected sand flies.

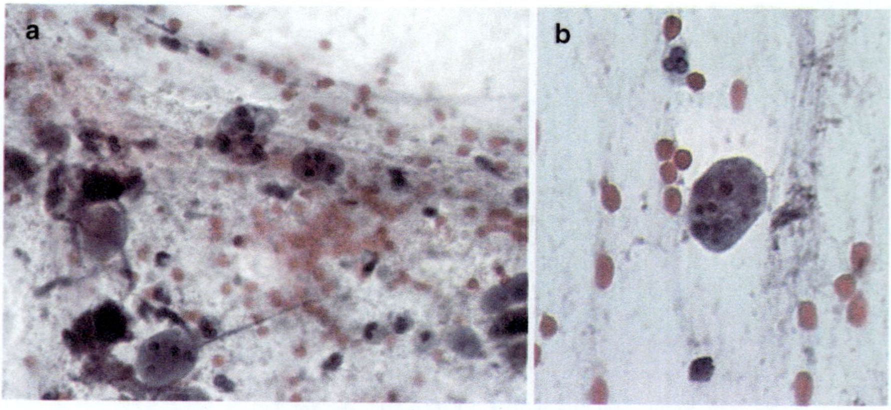

Fig. 4.3 (**a, b**) Smear showing Entamoeba gingivalis—with occasional epithelial cells and RBCs in inflammatory background

Mucocutaneous lesions of the oral cavity are caused by *L. braziliensis*. They present as moist ulcerating or nonulcerating lesions. The smears stained by Giemsa stain show a mixed inflammatory infiltrate along with the parasite (Donovan bodies) containing histiocytes, mononucleated, or binucleated (Reed-Sternberg-like) cells in association with lymphocytes, mast cells, and plasma cells [14, 15]. In late stages, it may become granulomatous. However, higher sensitivity is reported in FNAC smears as compared to scrape smears [16]. The parasites are rarely visible; eventually the lesion heals [17].

Entamoeba gingivalis: Entamoeba gingivalis is rarely seen in the lesions of the oral cavity [18], but it may be found in oral smears after radiation therapy and has been associated with periodontal disease [19] especially necrotic periodontal disease in immunocompromised patients [20]. The parasites look like histiocytes, with abundant cytoplasm, vesicular nucleus, a characteristic karyosome and pale blue biphasic granular cytoplasm containing basophilic fragments of cellular debris, stained with Giemsa, Trichrome or Gram stains (Fig. 4.3a, b) [21, 22]. A heavily inflamed background with numerous neutrophils may be present [18, 19, 23]. Other ancillary techniques may be used to detect these organisms [24].

Fungal Infections

Fungal infection is called mycosis. Fungi grow predominantly by budding (yeast) or by filamentous extensions called hyphae (molds). With rare exceptions, most fungi are diagnosed by cytology, by their morphology rather than staining characteristics. For their diagnosis, clinical observation plays an important role. They present as sore throat, ulcers or thrush in the oral cavity. The oral smears show hyphal or yeast forms which vary in size and shape. They present as budding, branching and sporangial forms. Sometimes, special stains, culture, or immunotechniques are used for identification of the fungus.

Candidiasis: Candidiasis is the most common opportunistic fungal infection of the oral cavity. Local and systemic factors can promote or enhance the development or sometimes, disseminate the disease [25]. It is mainly caused by Candida albicans, present in the oral cavity as a harmless commensal. It presents with pseudomembranous lesions—Candidiasis (Thrush), as smooth creamy white or yellow plaques. When these plaques are removed a red underline mucosa is seen. Erythematous Candidiasis (Atrophic)—presents as a red patch on the mucosa. Hyperplastic (Chronic) Candidiasis is recognized as non-removable whitish plaques [2]. The cytological diagnosis is made by the presence of long pseudohyphae or yeast forms in the oral smears [9]; Periodic acid Schiff (PAS) stain and Grocott Methenamine Silver stain (GMS) facilitate the detection of fungus both in hyphal and spore forms, along with acute inflammatory infiltrate [26]. In the PAS stain, it takes bright magenta color due to abundant carbohydrate in fungal cell walls. The infected epithelial cells exhibit nuclear enlargement, perinuclear rings, discrete orangeophilia, and cytoplasmic vacuoles (Fig. 4.4a–c). On cytomorphometry, the cytoplasmic area (CA) of the epithelial cells is diminished along with significant changes in size and shape of these cells [27]. In chronic infections, the smears may give false negative result [28], and then diagnosis is done by culture or employing ancillary techniques.

Paracoccidioidomycosis: It is a deep fungal infection caused by the dimorphic fungus—*Paracoccidioides brasilienesis*; it is seen as multiple mulberry-like ulcers on the oral mucosa, which can be confused with carcinoma and other infections like tuberculosis, histoplasmosis, and actinomycosis [29]. Oral exfoliative cytology can be a good tool for identification of these organisms especially when an invasive method is not indicated, especially in HIV patients [30]. The oral smears stained by Papanicolaou stain show round, birefringent multiple-budded fungi, lying free or in multinucleated giant cells and epithelioid cells, acute and chronic inflammatory cells, rich in neutrophils, along with the exosporulated forms of the fungi [2, 29, 31]. The yeast form varies from buds of 2–10 μm to cells up to 30 μm [32]. The organisms often show multiple daughter buds on the parent cell, resembling "Mickey-Mouse ears" or give a steering wheel appearance (Mariner's wheel). In case of negative results and persistence of strong clinical suspicion, ancillary techniques, or biopsy is advised to confirm the diagnosis [29].

Histoplasmosis: It is a systemic fungal infection caused by a dimorphic fungus—*Histoplasma capsulatum*, which is omnipresent, being endemic in the Ohio-Mississippi river valley in the USA [33, 34]. The lesion presents as a papillary, ulcerated, or nodular lesion involving the tongue, palate, and buccal mucosa, and sometimes mimicking malignancy [35]. Histoplasmosis is of clinical importance as it is frequently seen in immunosuppressed individuals, more often in HIV patients [36]. In oral lesions, exfoliative cytology is a useful tool for identification of the organisms, especially when invasive techniques are not indicated [37]. The oral smears show macrophages containing numerous intracellular small round or oval bodies, 1–5 μm yeast forms surrounded by a small light halo, in contrast to the spores of *H. duboisii*, which are much smaller [33]. Even the presence of a single budding yeast form is strongly suggestive, especially when found intracellularly—allowing immediate therapy. If required, the diagnosis can be confirmed by demonstrating the presence of specific anti-Histoplasma antibodies and culture.

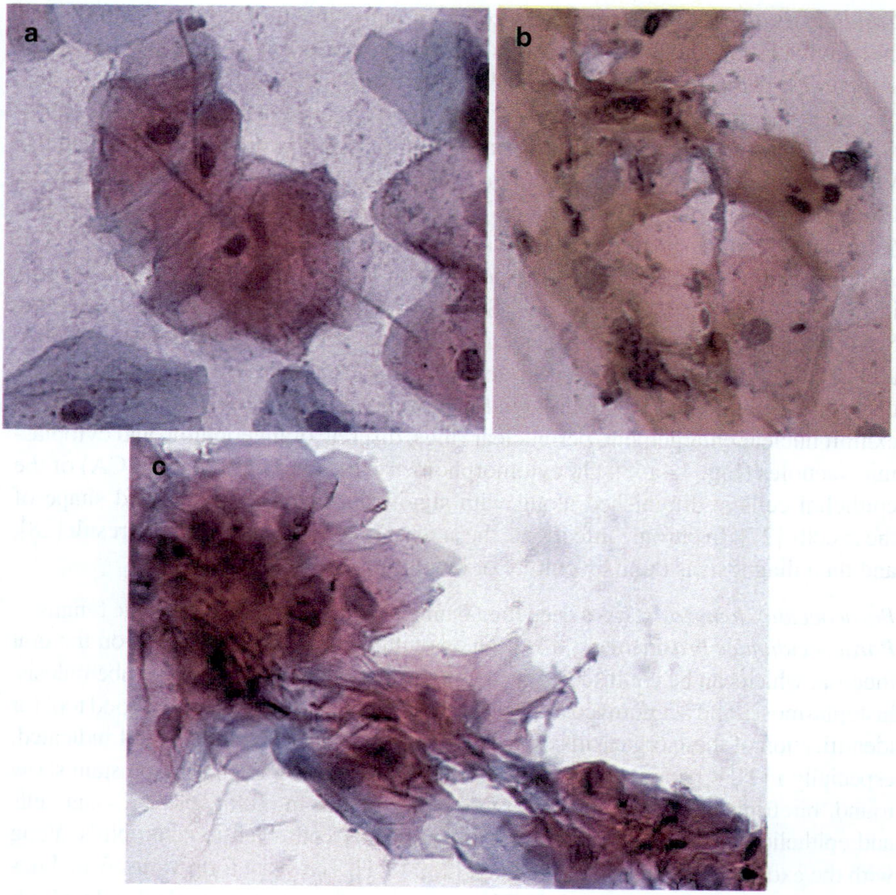

Fig. 4.4 (**a–c**) Epithelial cell showing evidence of Candidiasis

Cryptococosis: It is also present as a widespread infection and occurs by inhalation of spores present in the soil, rotting fruits and vegetables, excreta of birds like pigeons, canaries, and parrots. Infection is more common in immunocompromised patients and can involve skin, mucosa, lungs, meninges, bone, liver, and other tissues [38].

FNAC is a useful tool for rapid diagnosis of mucosal Cryptococcosis. The smears show a combination of acute inflammation and granuloma and can be confirmed by special stains for the fungus [39, 40]. The smears may show organisms of varying sizes—both intracellularly and extracellularly—in an acute or chronic granulomatous background [40]. In Hematoxylin and eosin (HE) stain, it looks like a bubble of 4–6 μ with a clear halo. A mucinous capsule of 3–5 μm can be seen by Mucicarmine and Alcian Blue (AB) staining. PAS and GMS stain the wall of the fungus but not the capsule. In Papanicolaou stain, it shows autofluorescence and gives quick results

[41]. Due to its typical morphology and inflammatory reaction, this fungus is easily recognized in the smears [2].

Aspergillosis: Aspergillosis can be caused by different species of *Aspergillus* but the most common is *A. fumigatus*. This fungus is a saprophyte and found in soil and decaying materials. It is an airborne infection through respiratory airways by inhalation of conidia (2–3 μm) and the hyphae. It causes necrosis and inflammation along with degenerated epithelial cells [42], especially in immunocompromised patients. In almost 68% cases of acute myeloid leukemia (AML) *Aspergillus* infection is seen in the oral cavity [43]. The lesion is seen in the palate, alveolar region and posterior tongue. It is characterized by yellow to black necrotic ulcers [44]. When the smears are stained by PAS and GMS, the fungus is seen as narrow nonseptate hyphae (2–7 μm); branching at an acute angle associated with conidiophores and conidia. Immunostains can help in quick diagnosis [45]. Sometimes, for final diagnosis, ancillary techniques are required.

Mucormycosis: It is also called Zygomycosis; it may cause fatal naso-cerebral infections which can damage the nasal septum, palate, maxilla, and the gingiva [46]. Infection occurs by inhalation of spores and also by ingestion or direct traumatic skin inoculation [47]. After inhalation the fungus reaches from the nose to paranasal sinuses, orbit, cribriform plate, and brain; the involvement of hard palate is less common [48].

Smears show large (5–50 μm), pleomorphic hyphae of irregular width (6–25 μm or more), with right angle dichomatously branching [49]. The twisted hyphae can look septated but rarely non-septated forms may be seen [50] along with an acute inflammatory infiltrate. For identification culture or immunostains are required.

Viral Infections

Viral infections are recognized by cytopathic effects in the epithelial cells in oral smears. These changes may be nonspecific or specific in the form of nuclear and/or cytoplasmic inclusions, indicating the causative organism. This may be accompanied with regenerative or reparative atypia along with cellular alterations. In cytologic preparations, few viruses can be recognized by specific cytomorphological changes, for example in measles infection, in addition to lymphocytes and macrophages, giant cells (Warthin-Finkeldey giant cells) may be seen in oral smears from the tonsillar area.

Herpes Viruses

Herpes simplex virus (HSV-1 and HSV-2): This is the most common viral infection of the oral cavity [51]. It is frequently found in young, sexually promiscuous or immunocompromised patients [52, 53]. After the infection, the virus may remain latent in neural tissues. Acute herpetic gingivostomatitis is the most common manifestation of

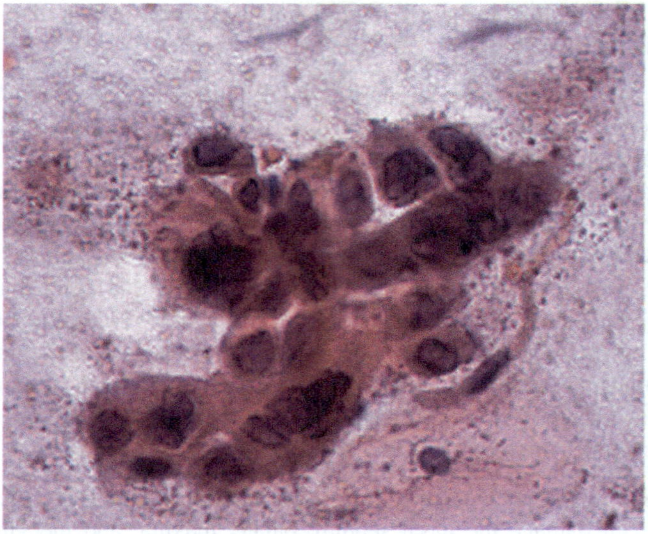

Fig. 4.5 Smear showing epithelial cells with eosinophilic cytoplasm, multinucleation, anisonucleosis, and thickening of nuclear membrane with ground glass appearance—Herpes virus infection

primary HSV-1 infection in children. This leads to severe gingivitis and vesicular lesions in the oral mucosa and may be associated with cervical lymphadenopathy.

The cytological presentation of HSV is better seen by Papanicolaou stain in comparison to Romanowsky stains. It includes binucleated and syncytial multinucleated giant cells along with ballooning of cytoplasm (Fig. 4.5) and Cowdry type A intranuclear eosinophilic inclusions with partial or complete loss of chromatin, these inclusions are separated from the thick nuclear membrane by a clear zone or halo. The cells show enlarged degenerated nuclei with smudged and homogenized ground glass and slate gray appearance (Cowdry B nuclei) [54]. HSV does not show intracytoplasmic inclusions; however, sometimes, subtle shading within the nucleus may be mistaken for inclusions. Similar changes may be seen in Cytomegalovirus infection—therefore, detection of HSV-1 genetic material is mandatory which may be done by the immunoperoxidase method [55]. Although routine stains provide indirect evidence for HSV infection, confirmation requires other tests like culture, immunocytochemistry, immunofluorescence, and in situ hybridization [56].

Cytomegalovirus (CMV): CMV belongs to herpes virus family and is also a problem in immunocompromised patients especially after renal transplant [57], frequently found with HSV in oral ulcers—this suggests a synergistic relationship [58].

CMV remains latent and may be reactivated in patients with low immunity status [59]. Then it manifests as painful ulcers and erosions on the lips, tongue and oral mucosa [60, 61]. In the smears, infected cells show both intracytoplasmic and intranuclear inclusions which can also be seen by both Papanicolaou and Diff Quick (DQ) stains. As its name, the size of infected cell increases remarkably. The nucleus shows prominent, often eosinophilic owl's-eye inclusions [62], with marginated chromatin that results in a halo effect and the cytoplasm shows numerous cytoplasmic inclusions—stained bright magenta color with DQ, easily visualized even at a scanning magnification. Sometimes, epithelial cells lack this characteristic finding and show small nuclear inclusions and incomplete round clear nuclear zone, or there may be binucleated, triangulated joint cells with inclusions like HSV-1 infection. Sometimes, the nuclear changes may be mistaken for malignancy [63]. Culture and molecular techniques may be used for final diagnosis [14].

Varicella Zoster virus (VZV): This infection may remain asymptomatic for years; disease occurs mainly in the elderly, children and immunosuppressed patients [64, 65]. It manifests as painful multiple vesicles on the facial skin, lips, and oral mucosa—usually along the root of trigeminal nerve and is diagnosed clinically. The oral lesions coalesce to form large ulcers which can also affect gingival and other parts of the oral cavity. This infection shows highly characteristic cytological changes in the form of multinucleation in epithelial cells with molding and clearing of the chromatin, prominent nuclear membranes; along with strong neutrophilic infiltration. Smears from the base of the lesions reveal multinucleated giant cells—Tzanck cells [14]. However, this technique cannot distinguish between HSV and VZV infection. For this, the smears may be examined by immunofluorescence. This technique is more sensitive than electron microscopy [66].

Molluscum contagiosum virus (MCV): Molluscum contagiosum is a disease caused by a poxvirus of the Molluscipox virus genus that produces a benign self-limited papular eruption of pearly white button-like, waxy or shiny multiple umbilicated lesions of the skin and mucous membranes. It is more prevalent in children with the lesions involving the face including oral cavity, trunk, and extremities. In adults the lesions are most often found near the genital region [67].

The oral scrape or FNAC smears can show nucleated and anucleated squames in an inflammatory background with Molluscum body—squamous epithelial cells with large, hyaline, acidophilic intracytoplasmic granular mass [14]. From the lesion, a thick white central core can be expressed and smeared on a slide and left unstained or stained with Giemsa, Gram, Wright, or Papanicolaou stains to demonstrate the large brick-shaped inclusion bodies [68]. Electron microscopy has also been used to demonstrate the poxvirus structures. Immunohistochemical methods using a polyclonal antibody allow recognition of Molluscum contagiosum in fixed tissue [69]. In situ hybridization for MCV DNA has also been utilized [70]. Molluscum contagiosum lesions must be differentiated from verruca vulgaris, condyloma acuminata, varicella, herpes simplex, papillomas, epitheliomas, pyoderma, cutaneous Cryptococcosis, epidermal inclusion cyst, basal cell carcinoma, papular granuloma annulare, keratoacanthoma, lichen planus, and syringoma or other adenexal tumors.

Epstein-Barr virus: This virus is a member of Herpes virus family and is present in 95% adult population of the world [71]. Usually it is asymptomatic, and manifests in immunocompromised patients suffering from diseases like HIV infection,

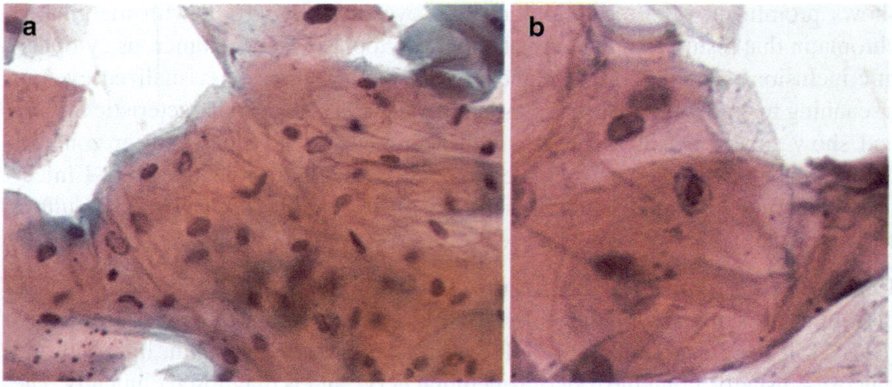

Fig. 4.6 Smear showing degenerative changes as cytoplasm vacuolization, thickening of nuclear membrane, ground glass appearance of the nuclear chromatin with inclusion bodies in inflammatory background—Epstein Barr virus infection

Hodgkin disease, lymphoma, malignancy, after chemotherapy, radiation, and patients on steroids. It may be seen in cases of oral hairy leukoplakia and other lesions of the oral cavity [72]. Clinically, it is seen as a white corrugated painless patch which is not easily scraped off, usually at the sides of tongue and mistaken for hyperkeratosis, pseudomembranous candidiasis, lichen-planus, oral white sponge nevus, and glossitis.

Oral smears show a nonspecific inflammatory infiltrate with nuclear changes suggestive of viral infection. Papanicolaou-stained smears show condensation and margination of the nuclear chromatin (nuclear beading) [73], sometimes Cowdry A inclusion bodies [72], usually inclusions are not seen in the infection, like HSV [9] (Fig. 4.6a–b). In biopsy specimens and in smears, koilocytes may display positive Epstein-Barr virus deoxyribonucleic acid in situ hybridization [74]. Final diagnosis is made by serological tests and advanced ancillary techniques [75].

Human herpes virus-8 (HHV-8): It is a member of γ-Herpes virus family and is the positive agent of Kaposi's sarcoma [76, 77]. Principally, it is transmitted sexually and sometimes through nonsexual routes also [78]. The virus is present in the saliva, causing oral lesions especially in immunocompromised patients in the form of patches, plaques and nodules [79]. The cytology show changes like other herpes viral infections. Smears, in such cases, show nuclear changes like Cowdry type A inclusions surrounded by a clear zone, homogeneous nuclear membrane with peripheral margination of chromatin and ground glass nuclei. However, the cytodiagnosis shows low sensitivity and specificity because these morphological changes are also seen in other viral infections. Therefore, for final diagnosis ancillary methods like immunocytochemistry [80], in situ hybridization, PCR [72] and electron microscopy are required [75, 81–82].

Respiratory viruses: They include a group of viruses like adenovirus, respiratory syncytial virus (RSV), influenza and para-influenza, and measles viruses. In adenovirus infection, cells show enlarged nucleus, containing amphophilic or basophilic inclusions and thin rim of cytoplasm smudge cells [83]. In measles infection, the changes have already been described. In RSV infection, epithelial cells show pink intracytoplasmic inclusions, often in a paranuclear location along with multinucleated giant cells [14]. It is very difficult to recognize these infections by oral cytology because the changes are not specific. The cytopathic changes of the epithelial cells include cytoplasmic eosinophilia with degenerative granules and vacuoles, nuclei show ground glass appearance of the chromatin; sometimes, forming giant cells. Laboratory investigations like viral culture, immunofluorescence and DNA probes are more reliable techniques for the diagnosis of these infections [83–85].

Human immunodeficiency virus (HIV): This virus infects the body sexually, by infected blood transfusion, mother to child transmission, by infected needles, and other routes. Acquired immunodeficiency syndrome (AIDS) is an infectious disease caused by the HIV, and is characterized by profound immunosuppression that leads to opportunistic infections, secondary neoplasm and neurologic manifestations.

Painful aphthous ulcers of unknown cause may occur in oral cavity. The smears on immunocytochemistry show an altered distribution of cytokeratin and may reflect local responses to proliferative stimuli by viral infection leading to proliferation of oral epithelial cells [86]. The oral smears show nonspecific inflammatory infiltrate or changes due to secondary infection by bacteria and fungi [9]. Final diagnosis is made by serology and ancillary techniques [9].

Human polyomavirus: Human polyomavirus is a member of papavaviridae family and is sporadically identified in urinary and other specimens. This may be seen in normal individuals and causes disease in immunosuppressed patients [54].

In oral infections, the solitary cells show enlarged nuclei with nuclear inclusions that almost fill the nucleus, leaving only a thin rim or halo—these large, opaque inclusions may be mistaken for malignant cells and therefore they have been termed as Decoy cells [87–89]. Due to their large size, they resemble CMV infection also. Immunodiagnostic techniques help to confirm the diagnosis.

Human Papilloma Virus (HPV): This is a non-enveloped, double-stranded DNA virus with more than 100 subtypes identified till date [90], constitutes the most widely prevalent sexually transmitted disease worldwide [91–94]. Diseases of the oral mucosa induced by HPV infection include oral verrucae vulgaris, squamous papillomas, Condylomata acuminata, Leukoplakia and focal epithelial hyperplasia (Heck's diseases) and neoplasia [95, 96].

Condylomata acuminata are relatively common benign lesions of the skin or mucosa of the oral cavity and anogenital region, more frequent in men, involving the tongue and floor of the mouth. HPV type 6 and 11 are most commonly associated viruses [97]. It can also present as squamous papillomas and oral verrucae—generally

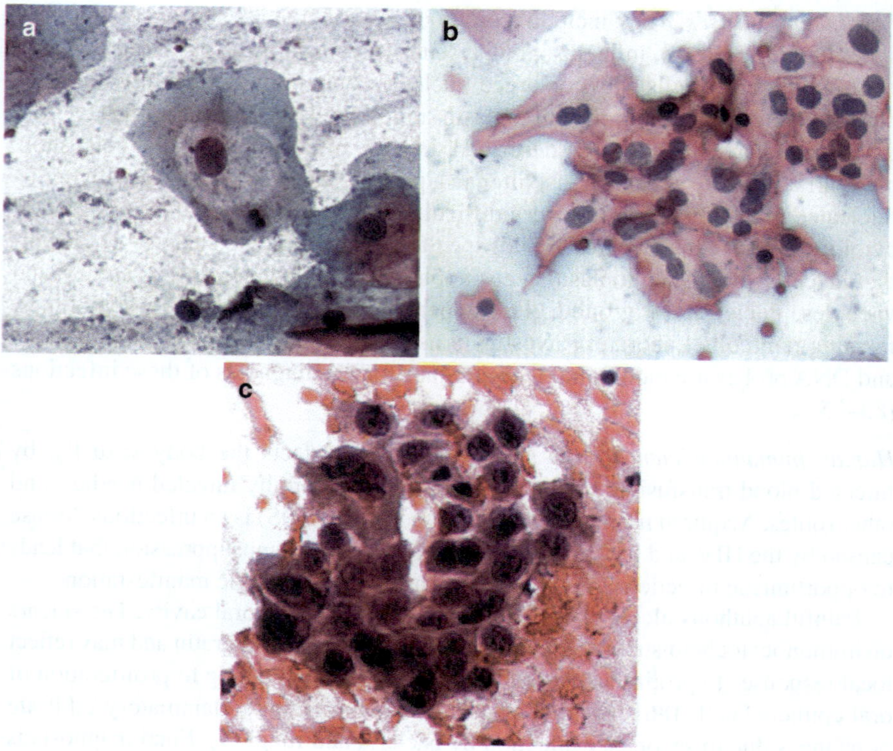

Fig. 4.7 (**a–c**) Clump of epithelial cells showing cytopathic changes due to viral infection (Human papilloma virus)—variation in cell size with localization of eosinophilic cytoplasm to the periphery, marked koilocytic change, anisonucleosis with hyperchromasia and binucleation (**a**, **b**) and dysplastic cells with multinucleation (**c**)

referred as oral warts seen on the oral mucosa and lips [91]. Rarely, focal epithelial hyperplasia is seen in HPV subtype 13 and 32. HPV can cause solitary or multiple lesions in any part of the oral cavity. The cellular hallmark in the epithelial cell is the koilocytic change [92]—characterized by peripheral margination of the cytoplasm with amphophilia, wrinkled nuclear membrane, perinuclear halo and binucleation and multinucleation of the cell—with or without dysplasia (Fig. 4.7a–c). HPV infection can be confirmed by PCR, ISH, and immunocytochemistry and by hybrid capture assay [93].

Cytopathic changes in the form of degenerating vacuoles, granules and koilocytic changes are pathognomic of HPV infection. The nucleus can show various types of atypia like anisonucleosis, thickening of the nuclear membrane, prominent nucleoli, inclusions, coarse chromatin; increased mitosis, etc. The dyskaryosis may range from mild to severe/carcinoma in situ and neoplasia [91].

Autofluorescence

Autofluorescence (AF) microscopy is a method whereby intrinsic fluorophore cellular molecules are excited by Ultraviolet/Light Emitting Diode (UV/LED) radiation of suitable wavelength, resulting in fluorescence emission and rendering these viewable by microscope. Auto-fluorescence should be distinguished from fluorescent signals obtained by adding exogenous markers [98].

The advantages of autofluorescence microscopy for oral and maxillofacial fungal and other pathogens screening include: no special staining procedures required—resulting in no time delays; the ability to screen material at a relatively lower power magnification and better pathogen discrimination against a dark background resulting in the ability to diagnose fungi (e.g., Candida, Aspergillus, Mucormycosis) with enhanced sensitivity (up to 97.8 %) and specificity (up to 100 %) [99–102]. However, there have been other reports that autofluorescence microscopy is of little benefit in identifying fungal organisms [103].

Autofluorescence microscopy is also widely used for the rapid diagnosis of mycobacterium infection [7, 104, 105]. Neethling and Wright have subjected smears containing a variety of organisms to LED fluorescent microscopy and observed that the following were positive: fungi (Candida, Aspergillus, Mucor, Pneumocystis, Cryptococcus, Histoplasmosis, Trichophyton); bacteria (*M. tuberculosis*, *M. leprae*, *M. bovis*, *Chlamydia*); protozoa, (Amoeba, Trichomonas); viruses (Molluscum), and other parasites (Echinococcus). These organisms showed various degrees of green to yellow fluorescence, highlighting the cell walls. The age of the specimens did not play a role in the strength of AF, as many cases were more than 10 years old. Actinomyces, Schistosoma and HPV-, HSV-, CMV-infected cells have been found to be negative for autofluorescence. They also confirmed that this technique is only effective on smears stained with the conventional, regressive PAP (CP) method, and not with the modified, rapid PAP (RP) staining method. It was concluded the AF is a rapid diagnostic modality ideal for use in immunocompromised patients, as it identifies three of the most common pathogens seen in AIDS patients i.e., Pneumocystis, Cryptococcus, and Mycobacterium spp. The advent of inexpensive LED fluorescent microscopy makes this technology affordable, especially, in resource limited countries [105].

Titinchi et al. similarly hypothesized that autofluorescence screening of Pap stained oral specimens may prove beneficial in cases where Candidal hyphae are otherwise undetected under normal light microscopy screening. Using AF in oral pathology and oral medicine practice may be a rapid screening test for subclinical candidiasis or the carrier state, specifically significant to Candidiasis associated with HIV infection and the early detection thereof in previously undiagnosed patients. Their study of double smears (respectively stained with Pap and PAS) from 80 patients cases revealed that both the Candidal hyphae and the oral squamous cells autofluoresce by the same color (Fig. 4.8a, b), thereby obscuring the detection of pathogens if either is superimposed (Fig. 4.9a, b) [106]. The same

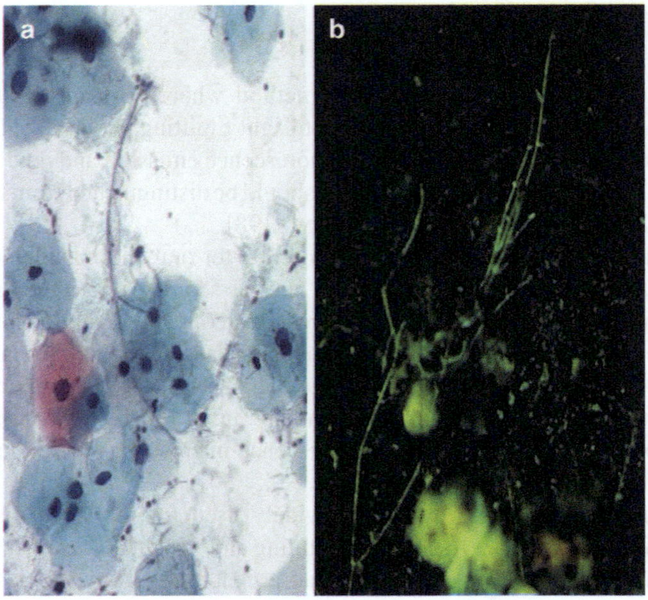

Fig. 4.8 (**a**) Squamous epithelial cells and septate, branching *Candida* spp. hyphae (Pap stain, ×400). (**b**) Autofluorescence of *Candida* spp. hyphae (LED/Pap stain, ×400). (Reprinted with permission, courtesy Titinchi et al. [106])

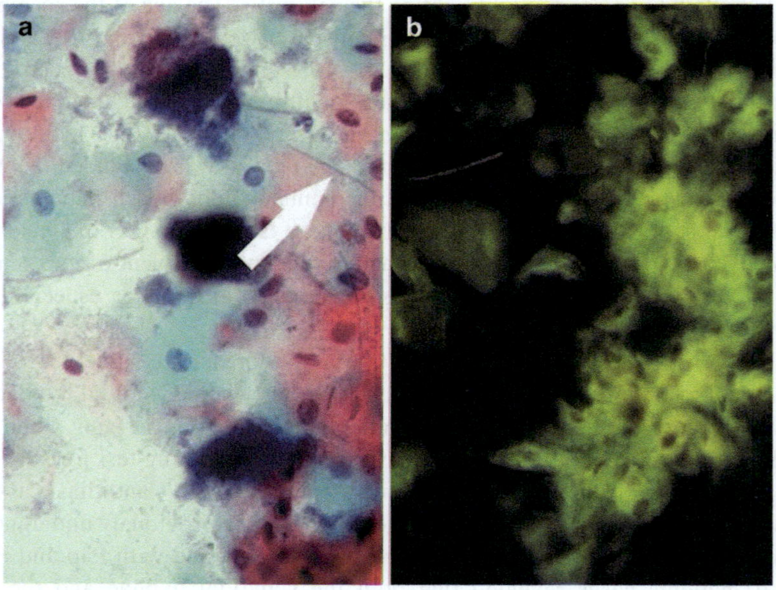

Fig. 4.9 (**a**) Squamous epithelial cells in close approximation to *Candida* spp. hyphus (*arrow*) (Pap stain, ×400). (**b**) The identical position within the same smear, autofluorescing squamous cells masking the fungus (LED/Pap stain, ×400) (Reprinted with permission, courtesy Titinchi et al. [106])

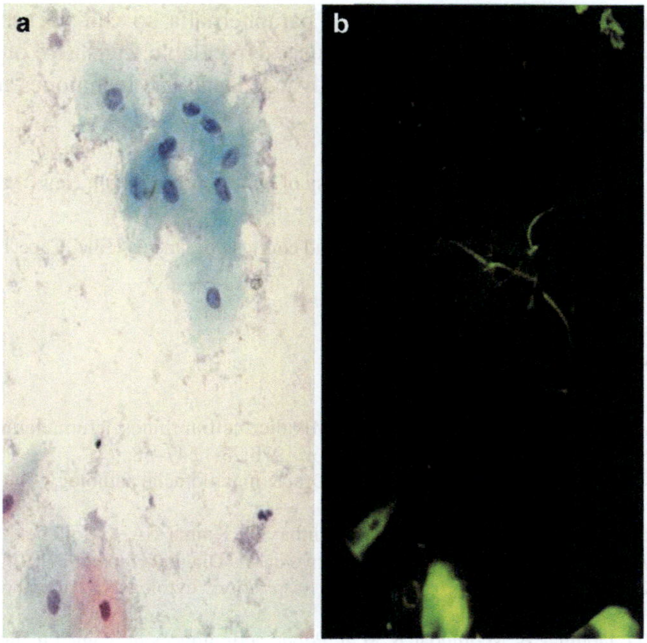

Fig. 4.10 (**a**) Possibly infected oral squamous epithelial cells (Pap stain, ×400). (**b**) The identical position within the same smear, squamous cells not autofluorescing and appearing as 'ghost cells' (LED/Pap stain, ×400) (Reprinted with permission, courtesy Titinchi et al. [106])

observation has been reported when examining cutaneous candidal infections using AF [103]. In such cases, it may be easier to detect hyphae using normal light microscopy. Conversely, hyphae not superimposed by squamous cells were rather distinct and easily detectable using LED/AF microscopy. It appears that Pap stained oral cytobrush material, viewed with LED/AF on its own, is not sufficiently effective/reliable when screening for oral Candida organisms. The orientation of the fungal hyphae in relation to the squamous cells may affect screening results significantly; pathogens detectable by autofluorescence microscopy may be otherwise undetectable by normal light microscopy, and vice versa. Periodic Acid Schiff (PAS)-stained oral smears viewed with normal light microscopy remains the gold standard with regards to identifying oral candidiasis or the carrier state. The two techniques may thus be deemed complimentary; possibly improving the accuracy of diagnosing candidiasis [106].

Finally, infection of squamous cells may possibly have a negative effect on their intrinsic ability to autofluoresce. In many cases oral squamous epithelial cells in close proximity to the fungal hyphae were visible under normal light microscopy (Fig. 4.10a), though interestingly appeared as 'ghost cells'—hidden when viewed under autofluorescence microscopy (Fig. 4.10b) [106].

In conclusion, oral cytology is often a good choice for identification of infective agents; being non invasive—therefore easily acceptable by patients, quick, cheap, simple, accurate, and requires minimum paraphernalia so can be used in mass screening especially in rural areas. Results are dependable; causative organisms of most of the lesions may be diagnosed and advanced ancillary techniques are required for final diagnosis in only a few cases.

Acknowledgements Figures 1–7 are kind courtesy of Dr. Deborah Carroll, New York.

The section on autofluorescence microscopy is kind courtesy of Dr. Jos Hille, Cape Town.

References

1. Hoffmann EO, Loose LD, Harkin JC. The Mikulicz cell in rhinoscleroma light, fluorescent and electron microscopic studies. Am J Pathol. 1973;73(1):47–58.
2. Brad WN, Douglas DD, Carl MA, Jerry EB. Oral & maxillofacial pathology. 2nd ed. Elsevier. 2005. p. 166–7.
3. Hemalata M, Prasad S, Venkatesh K, Niveditha SR, Kumar SA. Cytological diagnosis of actinomycosis and eumycetoma: a report of two cases. Diagn Cytopathol. 2010;38:918–20.
4. Das DK. Actinomycosis in fine needle aspiration cytology. Cytopathology. 1994; 5(4):243–50.
5. Hager WD, Douglas B, Majmudar B, et al. Pelvic actinomyces in women using intrauterine contraceptive devices. Am J Obset Gynecol. 1979;133:60–3.
6. Das DK, Bhatt NC, Khan VA, et al. Cervicofacial actinomycosis: diagnosis by fine-needle aspiration cytology. Acta Cytol. 1989;33:278–80.
7. Joshi P, Singh M, Bhargava A, Singh M, Mehrotra R. Autofluorescence—an important ancillary technique for the detection of Mycobacterium tuberculosis: revisited. Diagn Cytopathol. 2012. doi:10.1002/dc.21860. [Epub ahead of print]
8. Rees RJW. The microbiology of leprosy. In: Hastings RC, editor. Leprosy. Edinburgh: Churchill Livingstone; 1985. p. 31–52.
9. Kumar V, Abbas AK, Fausto N eds. Robbins and Cotran. Pathologic basis of Disease. 7th ed. Elsevier Saunders 2005. Pg. 193–26.
10. Alfieri N, Fleury RN, Opromolla DV, et al. Oral lesions in borderline and reactional tuberculoid leprosy. Oral Surg Oral Med Oral Pathol. 1983;55(1):52–7.
11. Smith WCS, Smith CM, Cree IA, et al. An approach to understanding the transmission of Mycobacterium leprae using molecular and immunological methods: results from the MILEP2 study. Int J Lepr Other Mycobact Dis. 2004;72(3):269–77.
12. Watanabe T, Matsuura M, Seto K. Enumeration, isolation, and species identification of mycoplasmasin saliva sampled from the normal and pathological human oral cavity and antibody response to an oral mycoplasma (Mycoplasma salivarium). J Clin Microbiol. 1986;23:1034–8.
13. Ned FK. Feline respiratory disease complex feline rhinotracheitis virus (FVR) and feline calicivirus (FVC). http://maxshouse.com/Resp_Di_.Comp.htm.
14. Woods GL, Walker DH. Detection of infection or infectious agents by use of cytologic and histologic stains. Clin Microbiol Rev. 1996;9:382–404.
15. Daneshbod Y, Oryan A, Davarmanesh M, et al. Clinical, histopathologic, and cytologic diagnosis of mucosal leishmaniasis and literature review. Arch Pathol Lab Med. 2011;135(4):478–82.
16. Hosseinzadeh M, Omidifar N, Lohrasb MH. Use of fine needle aspiration cytology in the diagnosis of cutaneous leishmaniasis: a comparison with the conventional scraping method. Trop Doct. 2012;42(2):112–3.

17. Chatterji KD. Parasitology protozoology and helminthology in relation to clinical medicine. 5th ed. Calcutta: Chatterjee Medical Publishers; 1980.
18. Perez-Jaffe L, Katz R, Gupta PK. Entamoeba gingivalis identified in a left upper neck nodule by fine-needle aspiration: a case report. Diagn Cytopathol. 1998;18:458–61.
19. Feki A, Molet B. Importance of Trichomonas tenax and Entamoeba gingivalis protozoa in the human oral cavity. Rev Odontostomatol (Paris). 1990;19:37–45.
20. Lucht E, Evengard B, Skott J, Pehrson P, Nord CE. Entamoeba gingivalis in human immunodeficiency virus type 1-infected patients with periodontal disease. Clin Infect Dis. 1998;27:471–3.
21. Garcia LS, Ash LRD. Diagnostic parasitology. St. Louis: Clinical Laboratory Manual C.V. Mosby Company; 1975.
22. Ghabanchi J, Zibaei M, Afkar MD, Sarbazie AH. Prevalence of oral Entamoeba gingivalis and Trichomonas tenax in patients with periodontal disease and healthy population in Shiraz, southern Iran. Indian J Dent Res. 2010;21:89–91.
23. Favoreto S Jr, Machado MI. Incidence, morphology and diagnostic studies of Entamoeba gingivalis, Gros, 1849. Rev Soc Bras Med Trop. 1995;28:379–87.
24. Kikuta N, Yamamoto A, Goto N. Detection and identification of Entamoeba gingivalis by amplification of rRNA gene. Can J Microbiol. 1996;42:1248–51.
25. Farah CS, Ashman RB, Challacombe SJ. Oral candidosis. Clin Dermatol. 2000;18:553–62.
26. Kayo Kuyama K, Sun Y, Taguchi C, et al. A clinico-pathological and cytological study of oral candidiasis. Open J Stomatol. 2011;1:212–7.
27. Loss R, Sandrin R, França BH, et al. Cytological analysis of the epithelial cells in patients with oral candidiasis. Mycoses. 2011;54:279–370.
28. Fitzhugh VA, Heller DS. Significance of a diagnosis of microorganisms on pap smear. J Low Genit Tract Dis. 2008;12:40–51.
29. de Araújo MS, Mesquita RA, Corrêa L, de Sousa SO. Oral exfoliative cytology in the diagnosis of paracoccidioidomycosis. Acta Cytol. 2001;45:360–4.
30. Luiz RT, Carlos PT. Paracoccidioidomycosis: advances in treatment incorporating modulators of the immune response. Int J Clin Rev. 2011; 05:08.
31. Cardoso SV, Moreti MM, Costa IM, Loyola AM. Exfoliative cytology: a helpful tool for the diagnosis of paracoccidioidomycosis. Oral Dis. 2001;7:217–20.
32. Almeida OP, Scully C. Fungal infections of the mouth. Braz J Oral Sci. 2002;1:19–26.
33. Cunha VS, Zampese MS, Aquino VR, Cestari TF, Goldani LZ. Mucocutaneous manifestations of disseminated histoplasmosis in patients with acquired immunodeficiency syndrome. Clin Exp Dermatol. 2007;32:250–5.
34. Kradin RL. Diagnostic pathology of infectious disease. Philadelphia; 2010.
35. Vishwanathan S, Chawla N, D'Cruz A, Kane SV. Head and neck histoplasmosis—a nightmare for clinicians and pathologists! Experience at a tertiary referral cancer centre. Head Neck Pathol. 2007;1(2):169–72.
36. Muñante-Cárdenas JL, de Assis AF, Olate S, et al. Treating oral histoplasmosis in an immunocompetent patient. J Am Dent Assoc. 2009;140(11):1373–6.
37. Muniz LB, Franco T, Ramos LM, et al. Oral exfoliative cytology in the diagnosis of histoplasmosis. Cytopathology. 2012;23:204–5.
38. Manfredi R, Calza L, Chiodo F. AIDS-associated Cryptococcus infection before and after the highly active antiretroviral therapy era: emerging management problems. Int J Antimicrob Agents. 2003;22:449–52.
39. Kumar P, Saran RK, Gondal R, Malhotra V. Smear morphology of cryptococcosis presenting as a subcutaneous swelling in healthy adults: a report of three cases. Cytopathology. 2005;16:143–6.
40. Srinivasan R, Gupta N, Shifa R, et al. Cryptococcal lymphadenitis diagnosed by fine needle aspiration cytology a review of 15 cases. Acta Cytol. 2010;54:1.
41. Nalini G, Rajwanshi A. Pulmonary infections. http://www.intechopen.com/download/pdf/32003.

42. Myoken Y, Sugata T, Kyo TI, et al. Pathological features of invasive oral aspergillosis in patients with hematologic malignancies. J Oral Maxillofac Surg. 1996;54:263–70.
43. Fuqua Jr TH, Sittitavornwong S, Knoll M, et al. Primary invasive oral aspergillosis: an updated literature review. J Oral Maxillofac Surg. 2010;68:2557–63.
44. Maiorano E, Favia G, Capodiferro S, et al. Combined mucormycosis and aspergillosis of the oro-sinonasal region in a patient affected by Castleman disease. Virchows Arch. 2005;446:28–33.
45. June-Ho B, Jeong-Hee L, Gyu-Jin R, et al. Squamous cell carcinoma occurring with aspergillosis in the maxillary sinus: a case report and histological study. J Korean Assoc Oral Maxillofac Surg. 2010;36:125–7.
46. Jones AC, Bentsen TY, Freedman PD. Mucormycosis of the oral cavity. Oral Surg Oral Med Oral Pathol. 1993;75(4):455–60.
47. Dave SP, Vivero RJ, Roy S. Facial cutaneous mucormycosis in a full-term infant. Arch Otolaryngol Head Neck Surg. 2008;134:206–9.
48. Barrak HA. Hard palate perforation due to mucormycosis: report of four cases. J Laryngol Otol. 2007;121:1099–102.
49. Julie AR, Carolyn LV. Zygomycetes in human disease. Clin Microbiol Rev. 2000;13(2):236–301.
50. Frater JL, Hall GS, Procop GW. Histologic features of zygomycosis. Emphasis on perineural invasion and fungal morphology. Arch Pathol Lab Med. 2001;125:375–8.
51. Whitley RJ, Roizman B. Herpes simplex virus infection. Lancet. 2001;357:1513–8.
52. Kapur S, Patterson K, Chandra R. Detection of herpes simplex infection in cytologic smears. Arch Pathol Lab Med. 1985;109:464–5.
53. Vernon SE. Cytologic features of nonfatal herpes virus tracheobronchitis. Acta Cytol. 1982;26:237–42.
54. Powers CN. Diagnosis of infectious diseases: a cytopathologist's perspective. Clin Microbiol. 1998;11(2):341–65.
55. Gupta RK, Buchanan AJ, Fauck R. Immunocytochemical confirmation of oral and respiratory herpesvirus infection by the immunoperoxidase method. Diagn Cytopathol. 1987;3(4):287–90.
56. Moseley RC, Corey L, Benjamin D, Winter C, Remington ML. Comparison of viral isolation, direct immunofluorescence, and indirect immunofluorescence techniques for detection of genital herpes simplex virus infection. J Clin Microbiol. 1981;13:913–8.
57. Abdallah PS, Mark JB, Merigan TC. Diagnosis of cytomegalovirus pneumonia in compromised hosts. Am J Med. 1976;61:326–32.
58. Regezi JA, Eversole LR, Barker BF, et al. Herpes simplex and cytomegalovirus co-infected oral ulcers in HIV-positive patients. Oral Surg Oral Med Oral Pathol Oral Radiol Endod. 1996;81(1):55–62.
59. Bloustein PA, Silverberg SG. Rapid cytologic examination of surgical specimens. Pathol Annu. 1977;12:251–78.
60. Ayre JE. Role of the halo cell in cervical cancerigenesis: a virus manifestation in premalignancy? Obstet Gynecol. 1960;13:735–8.
61. Brahic M, Haase AT. Detection of viral sequences of low reiteration frequency by in situ hybridization. Proc Natl Acad Sci USA. 1978;75:6125–9.
62. Wax TD, Layfield LJ, Zaleski S, et al. Cytomegalovirus sialoadenitis patients with the acquired immunodeficiency syndrome: a potential diagnostic pitfall with fine-needle aspiration cytology. Diagn Cytopathol. 1994;10:169–74.
63. Hilborne LH, Nieberg RK, Cheng L, Lewin KJ. Direct in-situ hybridization for rapid detection of cytomegalovirus in bronchoalveolar lavage. Am J Clin Pathol. 1987;87:766–9.
64. Quinlivan M, Breuer J. Molecular studies of Varicella zoster virus. Rev Med Virol. 2006;16:225.
65. Laboratory diagnosis of varicella zoster virus infections. http://virologyonline.com/viruses/VZV5.htm.
66. Kumar S, Siddaraju N, Mishra MM, Badhe BA, et al. Fine needle aspiration cytology of molluscum contagiosum. Acta Cytol. 2009;53:243–4.

67. Kumar N, Okiro P, Wasike R. Cytological diagnosis of molluscum contagiosum with an unusual clinical presentation at an unusual site. J Dermatol Case Rep. 2010;4(4):63–5.
68. Penneys NJ, Matsuo S, Mogollon R. The identification of molluscum infection of immunohistochemical means. J Cutan Pathol. 1986;13:97–101.
69. Thompson CH, Biggs IM, DeZwart-Steffe RT. Detection of molluscum contagiosum virus DNA by in-situ hybridization. Pathology. 1990;22:181–6.
70. Cheeseman SH, Henle W, Rubin RH, et al. Epstein-Barr virus infection in renal transplant recipients effects of antithymocyte globulin and interferon. Ann Intern Med. 1980;93(1):39–42.
71. Reginald A, Sivapathasundharam B. Oral hairy leukoplakia: an exfoliative cytology study. Contemp Clin Dent. 2010;1(1):10–3.
72. Migliorati CA, Jones AC, Baughman PA. Use of exfoliative cytology in the diagnosis of oral hairy leukoplakia. Oral Surg Oral Med Oral Pathol. 1993;76(6):704–10.
73. Kratochvil FJ, Riordan P, Auclair PL, Auclair PL, Huber MA, Kragel PJ. Diagnosis of hairy leukoplakia by ultra structural examination. Oral Surg Oral Med Oral Pathol. 1990;70:613–8.
74. Braz-Silva PH, Ortega KL, Rezende NP, Nunes FD, Magalhães MH. Detection of Epstein-Barr virus (EBV) in the oral mucosa of renal transplant patients. Diagn Cytopathol. 2006;34:24–8.
75. Braz-Silva PH, de Rezende NP, Ortega KL, de Macedo-Santos RT, de Magalhães MH. Detection of the Epstein-Barr Virus (EBV) by in situ hybridization as definitive diagnosis of hairy leukoplakia. Head Neck Pathol. 2008;2:19–24.
76. Martin JN, Ganem DE, Osmond DH, Page-Shafer KA, Macrae D, Kedes DH. Sexual transmission and the natural history of human herpesvirus 8 infection. N Eng J Med. 1998;338:948–54.
77. Widner IC, Erb P, Grob H, et al. Human herpesvirus 8 oral shedding in HIV-infected men with and without Kaposi sarcoma. J Acquir Immune Defic Syndr. 2006;42:420–5.
78. Webster-Cyriaque J, Edwards RH, Quinlivan EB, Patton L, Wohl D, Raab-Traub N. Epstein-Barr virus and human herpesvirus 8 prevalence in human immunodeficiency virus-associated oral mucosal lesions. J Infect Dis. 1997;175(6):1324–32.
79. Langford A, Kunze R, Schmelzer S, et al. Immunocytochemical detection of herpes viruses in oral smears of HIV-infected patients. J Oral Pathol Med. 1992;21:49–57.
80. Pauk J, Huang ML, Brodie SJ, et al. Mucosal shedding of human herpesvirus 8 in men. N Engl J Med. 2000;343:1369–77.
81. Mohammed MB, Hodgson TA, Cook RD, et al. Multiple human herpesvirus-8 infection. J Infec Dis. 2003;1885:678–89.
82. Walling DM, Flaitz CM, Adler-Storthz K, Nicholas CM. A non-invasive technique for studying oral epithelial Epstein-Barr virus infection and disease. Oral Oncol. 2003;13:436–44.
83. Johnston SL, Siegel CS. Evaluation of direct immunofluorescence, enzyme immunoassay, centrifugation culture, and conventional culture for the detection of respiratory syncytial virus. J Clin Microbiol. 1990;28:2394–7.
84. Matthey S, Nicholson D, Ruhs S, et al. Rapid detection of respiratory viruses by shell vial culture and direct staining by using pooled and individual monoclonal antibodies. J Clin Microbiol. 1992;30:540–4.
85. Dominguez EA, Taber LH, Couch RB. Comparison of rapid diagnostic techniques for respiratory syncytial virus and influenza A virus respiratory infections in young children. J Clin Microbiol. 1993;31:2286–90.
86. Langford A, Kunze R, Lobeck H, Pohle HD, Pl R. Distribution of cytokeratins in oral cytological smears of HIV-infected patients. J Oral Pathol Med. 1992;21(2):58–64.
87. Chappell LH, Lundin L. A pitfall in urine cytology: a case report. Acta Cytol. 1976;20:162–3.
88. Crabbe JG. "Comet" or "decoy" cells found in urinary sediment smears. Acta Cytol. 1971;15:303–5.
89. Akura K, Hatakenaka M, Kawai K, Takenaka M, Kato K. Use of immunocytochemistry on urinary sediments for the rapid identification of human polyomavirus infection. A case report. Acta Cytol. 1988;32:247–51.

90. Debnath S, Singh PA, Mehrotra R. Human papillomavirus infection and premalignant lesions of the oral cavity: a cross-sectional study in Allahabad North India. Asia Pac J Clin Oncol. 2009;5:111–8.
91. Singh M, Chaudhary AK, Pandya S, et al. Morphometric analysis in potentially malignant head and neck lesions: oral submucous fibrosis. Asian Pac J Cancer Prev. 2010;11(1):257–60.
92. Chaudhary AK, Pandya S, Mehrotra R, Bharti AC, Singh M, Singh M. Comparative study between the Hybrid Capture II test and PCR based assay for the detection of human papillomavirus DNA in oral submucous fibrosis and oral squamous cell carcinoma. Virol J. 2010;7:253.
93. Mehrotra R, Sharma N, Umudum H, Ceyhan K, Rezanko T. The role of cytopathology in diagnosing HPV induced oropharyngeal lesions. Diag Cytopathol. 2012;40(9):839–43.
94. Syrjänen S. Human papillomavirus (HPV) in head and neck cancer. J Clin Virol. 2005;32:59–66.
95. Nuovo GJ. Cytopathology of the lower female genital tract: an integrated approach. Baltimore: Williams and Wilkins; 1994.
96. Flaitz CM. Condyloma acuminatum of the floor of the mouth. Am J Dent. 2001;14:115–6.
97. Lynch DP. Oral viral infections. Clin Dermatol. 2000;18:619–28.
98. Monici M. Cell and tissue autofluorescence research and diagnostic applications. Biotechnol Annu Rev. 2005;11:227–56.
99. Mann J. Autofluorescence of fungi: an aid to detection in tissue sections. Am J Clin Pathol. 1983;79:587–90.
100. Wright CA, van der Burg M, Geiger D, Noordzij JG, Burgess SM, Marais BJ. Diagnosing mycobacterial lymphadenitis in children using fine needle aspiration biopsy: cytomorphology, ZN staining and autofluorescence – making more of less. Diagn Cytopathol. 2008;36:245–51.
101. Wright CA, van Zyl Y, Burgess SM, Blumberg L, Leiman G. Mycobacterial autofluorescence in Papanicolaou-stained lymph node aspirates: a glimmer in the dark? Diagn Cytopathol. 2004;30:257–60.
102. Rao S, Rajkumar A, Ehtesham M, Prathiba D. Autofluorescence: a screening test for mycotic infection in tissues. Indian J Pathol Microbiol. 2008;51:215–7.
103. Elston DM. Fluorescence of fungi in superficial and deep fungal infections. BMC Microbiol. 2001;1:21.
104. Subramony C, Cason Z, Gong JC, Evers CG. Fluorescence of Blastomyces and other fungi in Papanicolaou-stained pulmonary cytology preparations: comparison with light microscopy. Diagn Cytopathol. 1988;4:288–91.
105. Neethling G, Wright CA. Personal communication. 2012.
106. Titinchi F, Du Toit J, Hille J, Neethling G. The diagnostic accuracy of autofluorescence microscopy of Pap smears for oral candidal hyphae. Int J Oral Maxillofacial Pathol. 2011;2(4):28–33.

Chapter 5
Cytological Diagnosis of Benign Lesions of the Oral Cavity

Deborah J. Carroll

A review of the early history of oral cytopathology reveals mostly investigations into its sensitivity and specificity for detection of oral cancer [1–4]. The limited attention given to the cytopathology of benign oral conditions focused on its use for identification of either infectious agents or the characteristic cells in vesicubullous conditions such as pemphigus vulgaris [5, 6].

Interest in oral cytopathology as an instrument for cancer and precancer detection has increased in the last 15 years due to the emergence of new methods for obtaining and evaluating oral cytology specimens [7–17]. The introductions of sampling methods such as the brush biopsy, widespread use of liquid based technology, and capacity for evaluation of specimens using technology such as molecular analysis, cytomorphometry, and DNA cytometry have resulted in increased utilization of cytology to evaluate oral epithelium for evidence of dysplasia or cancer. One fortuitous consequence of this surge in interest in oral cytology has been the opportunity created to review and collect information not only about cancer and precancer, but also about a variety of benign oral conditions as well.

Benign lesions of the oral cavity can be divided into surface mucosal lesions, submucosal lesions, and jaw lesions of odontogenic or non-odontogenic origin [18]. Oral exfoliative or brush biopsy cytopathology generally affords an opportunity for evaluation only of surface mucosal or epithelial lesions. In the event of surface trauma or ulceration, however, cytopathologic evidence of non-epithelial processes may be detected.

D.J. Carroll (✉)
Oral CDx Laboratories, 2 Executive Boulevard, Suite 102, Suffern, NY 10901, USA
e-mail: dcarroll@cdxlabs.com

R. Mehrotra (ed.), *Oral Cytology: A Concise Guide*, DOI 10.1007/978-1-4614-5221-8_5,

Table 5.1 Color of lesions sampled January 2008–October 2011 Oral CDx Laboratories

Color	Number reported
White	43,591
Red	10,457
Mixed	13,661
Brown, "Pigmented", Black	386
Other, or not specified	7,557
Total	75,652

From an Oral CDx Laboratories (Suffern NY) case database query, unpublished results [22]

White Lesions

Benign white lesions of the oral mucosa can result from thickened keratin layer, epithelial hyperplasia, intercellular edema, diminished vascularity of subepithelium, fibrinous exudates, surface debris, fungus, or submucosal deposits [18]. Some will prove to have a definite identifiable cause; the remainder are classified as leukoplakias. Leukoplakia is a clinical term defined as a white patch or plaque not less than 5 mm in diameter which cannot be removed by rubbing and cannot be classified as any other diagnosable disease [19]. Histologically, over 80% of leukoplakias are benign lesions with hyperorthokeratosis, hyperparakeratosis, and acanthosis [20]. White oral lesions including leukoplakias are the most common lesions detected during oral screenings [21] and are the most common reason for oral cytopathologic evaluation. Of the greater than 75,000 oral brush biopsies seen at the OralCDx Laboratory between January 2008 and October 2011 more than half were clinically identified as samples of white lesions (Table 5.1).

Hyperkeratosis

Normal oral mucosa is non-keratinized stratified squamous epithelium and lacks a granular layer, except for the dorsal tongue, outer gingiva, and hard palate which are normally keratinized and the hard palate which may possess a granular layer [23]. Oral squamous mucosa has the capacity to exhibit only a limited range of potential reactive responses to epithelial injury or other stimuli promoting change; oral hyperkeratosis represents the most common. Hyperkeratosis is associated with numerous underlying oral conditions: 21% of lesions detected in one large series were keratotic, with leukoplakia being the most common diagnosis [24]. It is, of course, the association with dysplasia and squamous cell carcinoma in 5–20% of leukoplakias which prompts the greatest clinical concern when a white lesion is identified [19, 24, 25].

In smears from hyperkeratotic lesions it is important to distinguish benign hyperkeratosis from atypical hyperkeratosis which should prompt scalpel biopsy evaluation. The typical benign hyperkeratosis will show small parakeratotic cells with pyknotic nuclei, and anucleate single cells with non-refractive pink, yellow, or orange cytoplasm. Plaques of anucleate cells may be present, appearing more frequently as the thickness of the hyperkeratotic layer and the vigor of sampling increase. Also identified are parakeratotic sheets or strips with pink or orange cytoplasm and small, elongate or oval pyknotic nuclei with uniform nuclear spacing and orderly nuclear "streaming". Cells with cytoplasmic granulosis resembling that in the normal prickle cell layer of skin are frequently present.

In contrast, hyperkeratosis which should prompt a scalpel biopsy evaluation shows a greater number of single cells with anisonucleosis, nuclear hyperchromasia, with retention of chromatin granularity, and parakeratotic tissue fragments exhibiting apparently random nuclear orientation and irregular spacing with alternating areas of crowding and "empty" keratin (Fig. 5.1a–e).

Frictional Keratosis

A common etiology of an oral white lesion is focal or frictional keratosis resulting from trauma, such as that associated with tongue or cheek biting or ill-fitting dentures [26, 27]. Lesions shown histologically to be consistent with frictional keratosis present with cytology showing the features of benign hyperkeratosis as described above and illustrated in Figure 5.1. Inflammatory nuclear changes are not a prominent component.

Smokeless Tobacco Keratosis

The histopathologic changes in oral mucosa caused by smokeless tobacco have been described previously, the primary findings in benign lesions being hyperorthokeratosis, hyperparakeratosis, pale staining of surface cells, and basal cell hyperplasia [28–30]. Many of these lesions have a size of 20 mm or more. One advantage of oral cytopathology in the evaluation of these lesions is the ability to sample a wider area in one specimen than with a scalpel biopsy [5, 7]. The cytopathology of these lesions, especially those associated with the use of snuff is unique: so much so that the clinical history of smokeless tobacco use can in some cases be predicted, based on examination of the oral smear. Unlike other forms of oral keratosis, brush biopsy sampling of smokeless tobacco lesions produces a predominance of anucleate keratinocytes with numerous large keratin plaques, showing a variable combination of ghost nuclei, nuclear karyorrhexis, and cytoplasmic granulation ranging from fine and sparse to heavy and

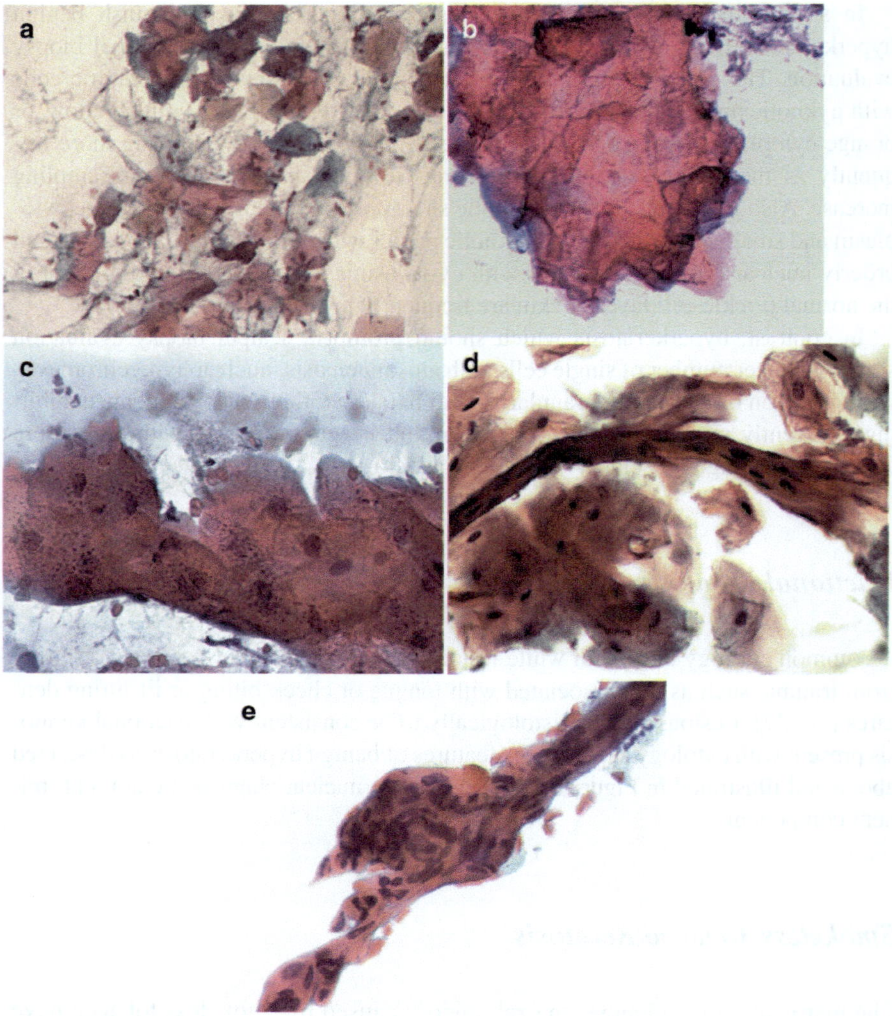

Fig. 5.1 Features of benign keratotic lesions: (**a**) Anucleate keratinocytes. (**b**) Anucleate plaque. (**c**) Cytoplasmic granulation reminiscent of that seen in the granular cell layer of skin. (**d**) Benign parakeratotic tissue fragment with oval nuclei and orderly nuclear streaming. (**e**) To contrast with benign parakeratosis, a tissue fragment showing atypical parakeratosis with variable nuclei, crowding and haphazard arrangement

coarse. Cytoplasmic staining may be orangeophilic or eosinophilic as in other types of hyperkeratosis, it may be biphasic, or it may more closely resemble that of intermediate cells—appearing blue or green. Many of these features have been described previously [31]. "Broken egg" nuclei may be present, but this finding is non-specific, appearing in other hyperkeratotic and reactive conditions (Fig. 5.2a–g).

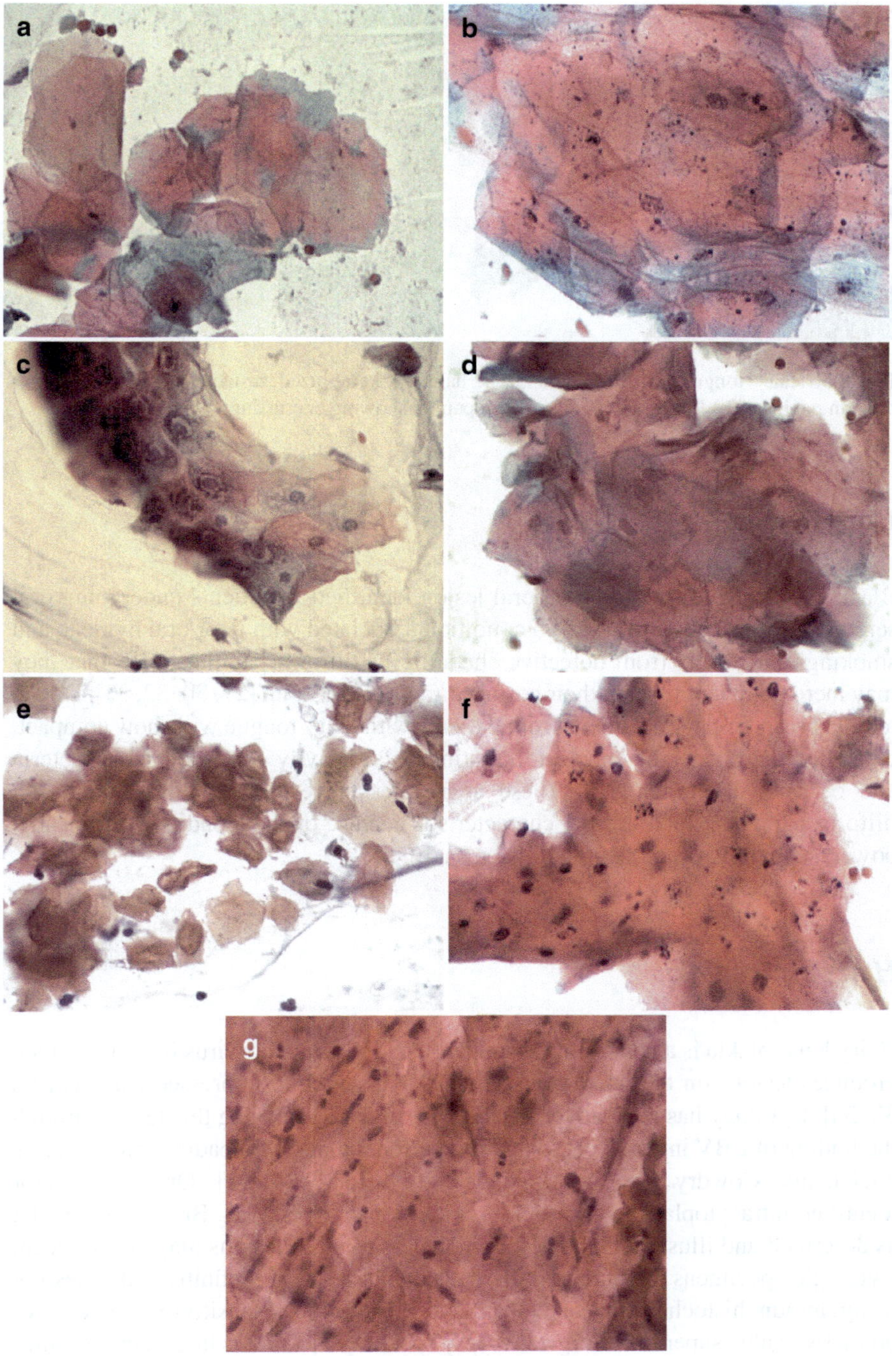

Fig. 5.2 Features of smokeless tobacco keratosis: (**a**) Biphasic anucleate plaques. (**b**) Sparse cytoplasmic granulation. (**c**) Coarse cytoplasmic granulation. (**d**) Pale staining of superficial cell nuclei. (**e**) Ghost nuclei. (**f**) Nuclear karyorrhexis. (**g**) Broken-egg nuclei

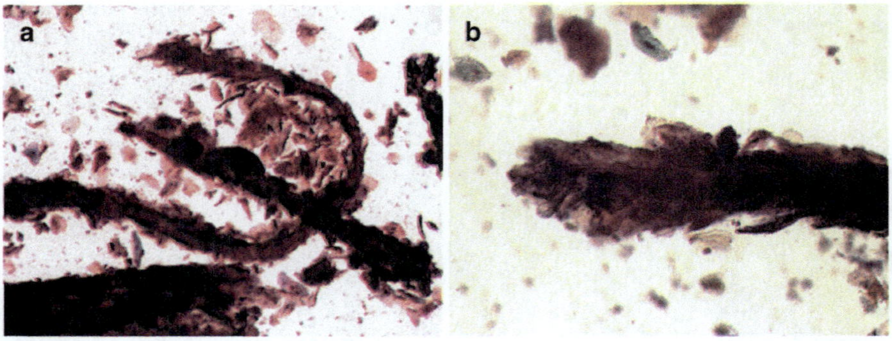

Fig. 5.3 Hairy tongue: (**a**) Brown to black hair-like keratinized structures corresponding to filiform papillae. (**b**) Higher power of filiform papilla showing encrusting with bacteria

Hairy Tongue

Black hairy tongue is a common oral lesion identified in patients undergoing oral screening examination [21]. It is a condition associated with poor oral hygiene and smoking and results from defective shedding of filiform papillae, such that they may increase in length from their normal 3 mm up to 15 mm [27, 30, 32, 33]. Dorsal tongue brush biopsy specimens from patients with hairy tongue will show compact, elongated aggregates of anucleate keratinocytes, heavily encrusted with bacteria and occasionally fungi [32]. These aggregates correspond to the hyperplastic filiform papillae which are the characteristic feature of this condition and at low power, strikingly resemble hairs (Fig. 5.3a, b).

Hairy Leukoplakia

Hairy leukoplakia is a condition associated with Epstein-Barr virus infection which produces lesions on the lateral tongue usually in immunosuppressed patients [27, 32, 34]. Cytology has been advocated as a means of identifying this lesion through the finding of EBV infected cells showing peripheral nuclear beading, ground glass nuclei, and Cowdry type A intranuclear inclusions [34, 35]. One investigator identified intracytoplasmic eosinophilic inclusions as well [36]. Broken egg nuclei as described and illustrated above for smokeless tobacco lesions may also be seen. Cytologic specimens have been utilized to obtain cells for definitive EBV testing using immunohistochemistry and in situ hybridization with sensitivity and negative predictive value superior to surgical biopsy specimens [37]. It is important to distinguish this condition from black hairy tongue because of the strong association with underlying HIV infection and concurrent or subsequent progression to AIDS [18]. Figure 5.4a–c.

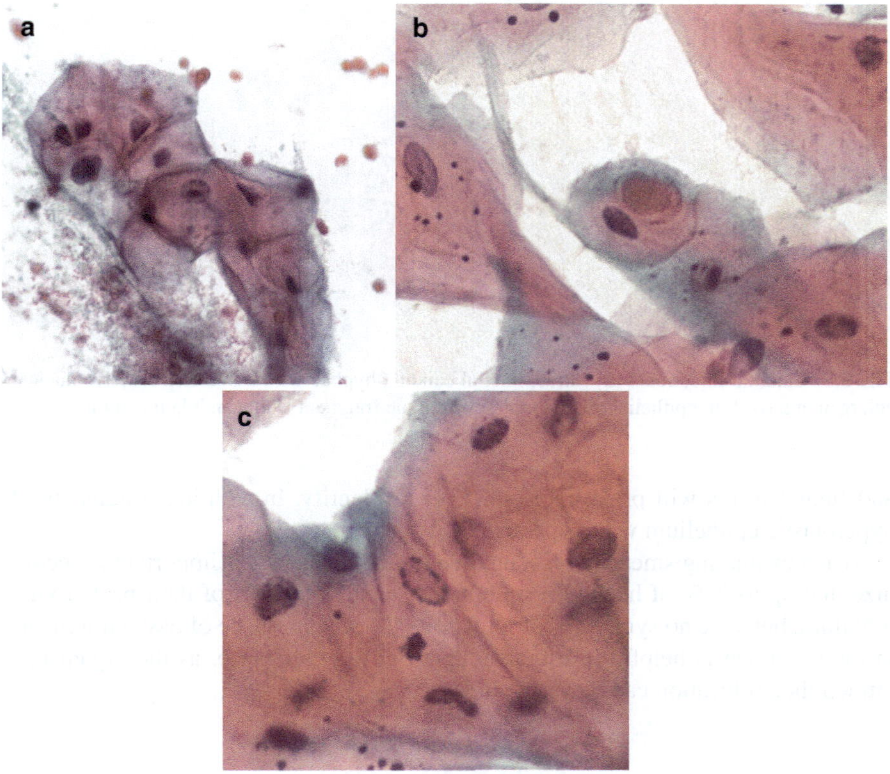

Fig. 5.4 Hairy leukoplakia: (**a**) Cowdry type A intranuclear inclusion. (**b**) Eosinophilic cytoplasmic inclusion. (**c**) Peripheral beading of chromatin

Candidiasis

Oral candidiasis is a common lesion—in one large study accounting for 78% of all lesions examined [38]. Oral candidiasis may have a variety of clinical appearances ranging from the white lesions of acute pseudomembranous candidiasis (thrush) and chronic hyperplastic candidiasis to the red lesions of angular cheilitis and chronic atrophic candidiasis (denture stomatitis) [39]. Infections predominate in persons with risk factors such as smoking, diabetes, immunosuppression, impairment of salivary gland function, and importantly, use of dentures. Chronic atrophic candidiasis may occur in up to 65% of elderly denture wearers [39].

In addition to the characteristic yeast and pseudohyphae, white lesions of acute candidiasis will typically show smears with reactive changes including benign hyperkeratosis, cells with nuclear enlargement, perinuclear rings, cytoplasmic vacuoles, and acute inflammation [40]. Tissue fragments with microabscesses may be present, as seen in histopathologic sections [18]. White lesions of chronic hyperplastic candidiasis may show similar changes, but inflammation will be less intense

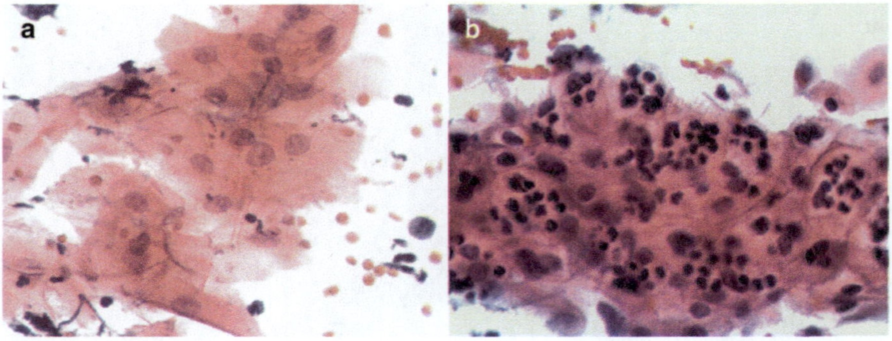

Fig. 5.5 Candida infections: (**a**) Intraepithelial candida hyphae with associated reactive nuclear enlargement. (**b**) Intraepithelial microabscesses in tissue fragment from candida infection

and fungal forms will prove more difficult to identify. In addition, fragments of hyperplastic epithelium will be present.

When evaluating smears with fungal yeast and hyphae, it is important to recognize that up to 75% of healthy people harbor candida as part of their background oral flora, but have no symptoms of infection [40]. The presence of tissue fragments in the specimen is helpful in establishing clinical significance, as the organism's intraepithelial location can be verified (Fig. 5.5a, b).

Fordyce Granule/Ectopic Sebaceous Gland

Fordyce granules or ectopic sebaceous glands are reportedly present in up to 80% of the population and can be considered a variant of normal [18]. Presenting usually on the buccal mucosa or vermilion border of the lip as white-yellow nodules, they are usually readily diagnosed clinically. Because they are located in the subepithelial space and lack a direct connection to the epithelial surface, evidence of Fordyce granules will generally be apparent only in specimens subjected to vigorous sampling or in specimens taken after surface trauma. Cytopathologic specimens will reveal scattered aggregates of cells with cytoplasm containing the characteristic small vacuoles corresponding to lipid droplets and closely resembling those seen in sebaceous lobules in surgical biopsy specimens (Fig. 5.6a, b).

Lymphoid Hyperplasia/Lymphoepithelial Cyst/Ectopic Lymphoid Tissue

Some white lesions will prove to be lymphoid tissue on surgical biopsy. Ectopic lymphoid tissue presents clinically as a small yellow or yellow white dome-shaped mucosal elevations [17]. Brush biopsy sampling will produce smears showing

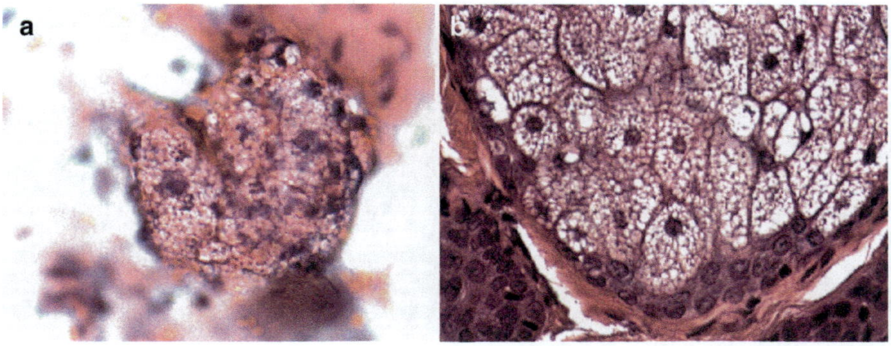

Fig. 5.6 Fordyce granule: (**a**) Vacuolated cells from brush biopsy of Fordyce granule. (**b**) Histology of Fordyce granule showing sebaceous lobule closely resembles cytology

benign squamous cells and a polymorphous lymphoid infiltrate aggregates with tingible body macrophages, an appearance similar to that seen in smears from chronic lymphocytic cervicitis [44].

If the crypts within one of these benign lymphoid aggregates or accessory tissue foci become obstructed, a lymphoepithelial cyst may be formed. Histopathologically, these are lined by atrophic and degenerated stratified squamous epithelium, with luminal orthokeratin [41–43]. Smears will show a mucoid background with lymphocytes and cyst contents consisting of small parakeratotic cells and anucleate keratinocytes, many showing indistinct cell borders and cytoplasmic fragmentation (Fig. 5.7a, b).

Vesiculobullous Lesions

Herpes Virus Infection

One of the classical uses of oral cytology has been for the evaluation of vesiculobullous lesions [5, 45]. Oral lesions caused by viruses of the Herpesvirus family present initially with vesicles which rupture, leaving painful ulcers [26, 46, 47]. Oral smears will demonstrate cells with viral cytopathic effect including multinucleation, ground glass nuclei, and nuclear molding identical to that seen in cervical smears [23, 48–50]. Intranuclear inclusions surrounded by a clear halo may be seen in well-preserved smears, but are more infrequent [45]. The typical background will demonstrate fibrinopurulent exudate, inflammation, blood, and tissue fragments with cytopathologic features of repair, consistent with ulceration. It should be noted that while the majority of oral Herpes virus lesions will be caused by Herpes simplex virus type 1 (or occasionally type 2), Herpes zoster may present with oral lesions [51] and it is not possible to differentiate cells infected with Herpes simplex virus from those infected by Varicella zoster virus using cytomorphology alone [45, 46, 51] (Fig. 5.8a, b).

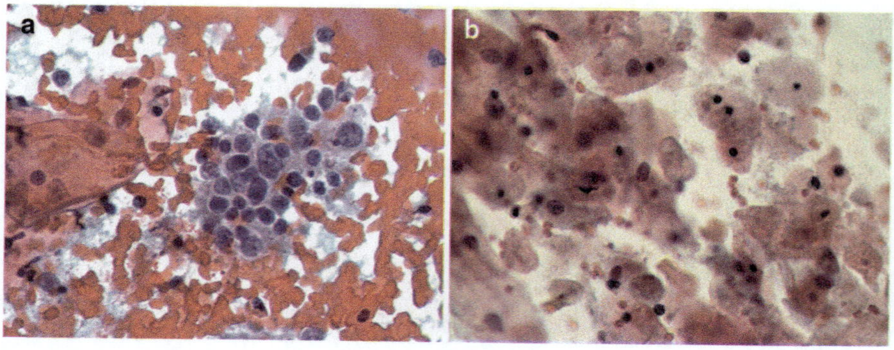

Fig. 5.7 Lymphoid tissue and lymphoepithelial cyst: (**a**) Benign lymphoid aggregate from brush biopsy of ectopic lymphoid tissue. (**b**) Lymphocytes and anucleate and parakeratotic cells with cytoplasmic degeneration from brush biopsy of lymphoepithelial cyst

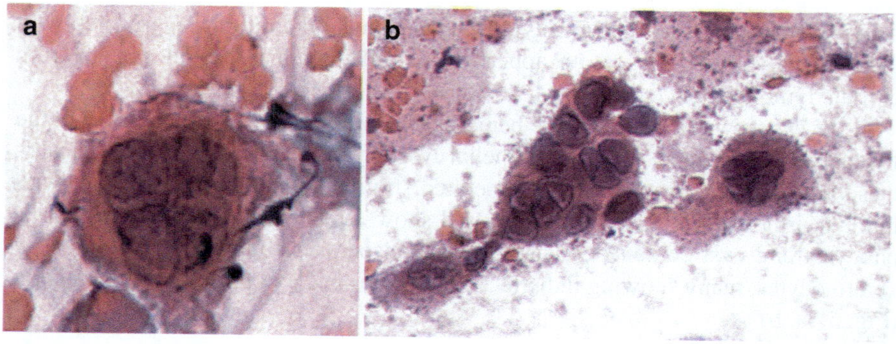

Fig. 5.8 Herpes virus infection: (**a**) Classic multinucleated cell with ground glass nuclei and nuclear molding in herpes virus infection. (**b**) Less common presentation with infected cells showing intranuclear inclusions with surrounding clear halo

Pemphigus Vulgaris

Pemphigus vulgaris is a chronic autoimmune intraepithelial blistering disease. It almost always affects the mouth and can be the initial site of presentation in 50% of cases before skin and other mucosal sites. It may present clinically as chronic mucosal ulceration of unknown cause [52, 53]. Patients with oral manifestations of pemphigus vulgaris have autoantibodies against desmosomes, specifically desmoglein 3 [52]. Lesions present as fluid filled blisters which rupture to form erosions.

In a well-preserved specimen, pemphigus vulgaris will demonstrate a moderately discohesive and relatively uniform population of basal and parabasal polygonal cells with accentuation of the nuclear membrane and nuclear clearing with prominent single or multiple nucleoli. Cytoplasm shows degeneration with wispy cytoplasmic extensions outward from the cell [49]. Intracytoplasmic vacuoles may also be present. Cytoplasm is often basophilic, but may vary relative to the degree of degeneration, sometimes appearing amphophilic [6]. Multinucleation may occur.

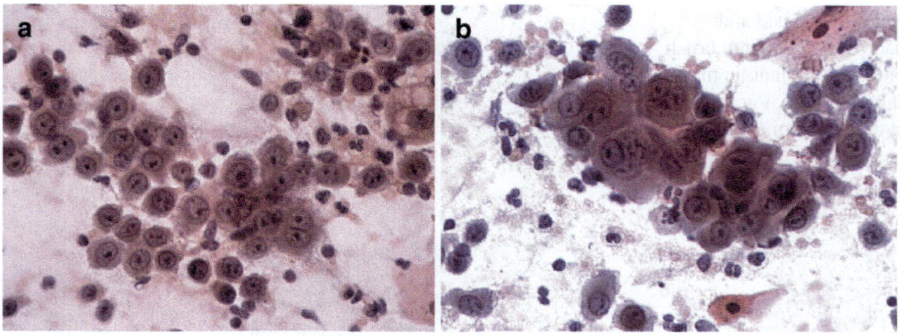

Fig. 5.9 Pemphigus vulgaris: (**a**) Acantholytic cells with cytoplasmic degeneration, nuclear membrane accentuation, and prominent nucleoli. (**b**) Multinucleation

Background features may include obscuring acute inflammation and blood with fibrinopurulent exudate, consistent with ulceration. Cytology smears showing changes consistent with pemphigus have been de-stained in ethyl alcohol and treated with immunocytochemical stains to render a definitive diagnosis of pemphigus vulgaris with cytology alone [54]. Figure 5.9a, b.

Pigmented Lesions

Because both benign and malignant pigmented lesions in the oral cavity typically have pathology critical to the diagnosis in the subepithelial space, cytopathologic specimens are not satisfactory for comprehensive evaluation of these lesions. Brush biopsy specimens can, however, prove useful in the evaluation of two conditions which present clinically as pigmented lesions: the melanotic macule and the amalgam tattoo.

Melanotic Macule

Oral melanotic macules usually present on the gingiva or lips in the fifth decade of life. Lesions are usually less than 1 cm and may be multiple. The melanin pigment in the melanotic macule resides not only in melanocytes but also in the parabasal and basal epithelial cells [55–57], so a deep brush biopsy specimen with tissue fragments including these cells may reveal melanin pigment in the cell cytoplasm. While it is reasonable to state that a specimen shows changes suggesting the lesion tested is a melanotic macule, cytology should not be utilized as the sole procedure for evaluation of pigmented oral lesions. The current recommendation is to excise all oral melanocytic lesions for histopathologic evaluation [55–57]. Figure 5.10.

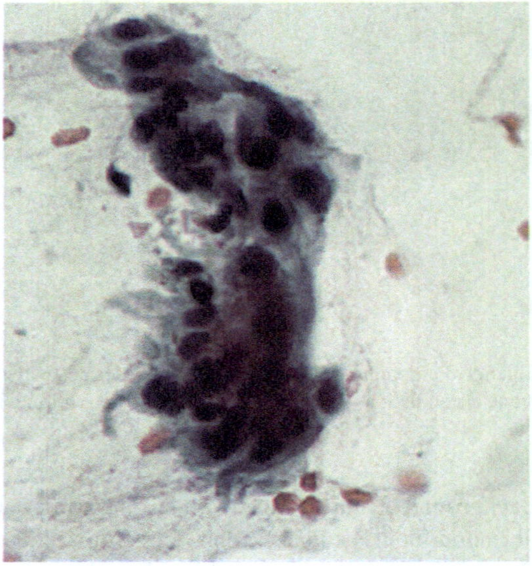

Fig. 5.10 Basal and parabasal cells from brush biopsy of melanotic macule showing brown granular cytoplasmic pigment

Amalgam Tattoo

Amalgam tattoo is the most common oral pigmentation, presenting clinically as a flat, gray discoloration of the oral mucosa. They are typically located in gingival or buccal mucosa, palate, and tongue near amalgam restorations. The cause is either inadvertent implantation of amalgam during restoration or chronic contact with an adjacent amalgam restoration [57]. The implanted amalgam has an affinity for subepithelial collagen fibers and blood vessels elastin, so superficial cytology specimens may reveal no distinguishing features. In brush biopsy specimens resulting from vigorous sampling, however, rare amalgam fragments may be evident. Amalgam appears as amorphous, black material, with slight translucency. The typical appearance is illustrated in Fig. 5.11a, an image taken from a smear made by mixing amalgam fragments with saliva.

Sometimes amalgam fragments will appear in a smear when the sample is taken in the same visit after a dental restoration is performed, but have no causal association with the lesion being sampled. The large number and size of the fragments in the smear, and the absence of correlating clinical history of a flat gray mucosal macule will prevent the erroneous conclusion that the specimen is taken from an amalgam tattoo (Fig. 5.11 b).

Subepithelial Processes

Generally, common oral lesions which are predominately subepithelial cannot be reliably sampled with oral brush biopsy or exfoliative cytology. If, however, there has been some disruption of the overlying epithelium either due to local trauma or to vigorous sampling technique, the occasional brush biopsy sample will reveal evidence of a subepithelial process. Subepithelial processes that have been sampled

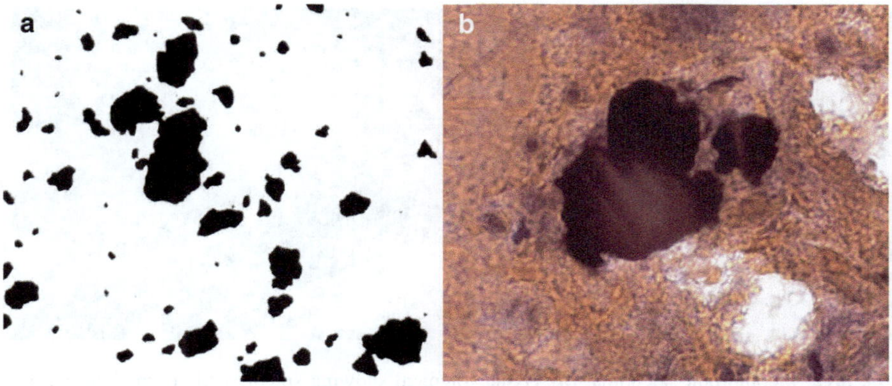

Fig. 5.11 Amalgam tattoo: (**a**) Saliva smear to illustrate amorphous, black, slightly translucent fragments of amalgam. (**b**) Amalgam fragment in brush biopsy from amalgam tattoo. Note bloody background indicating trauma

with the brush biopsy include fibromas, salivary gland tumors, Fordyce granules (described above), ameloblastoma, and mucocele.

Salivary Gland Tumors

The most common benign minor salivary gland tumor in the oral cavity is the pleomorphic adenoma and the most common location (over 50%) is the palate [58, 59]. Tumors typically present in the sixth decade of life, but have been reported in children [60]. Evaluation of the major salivary glands using cytopathology specimens obtained through fine needle aspiration has been well established. Evaluation of intra-oral salivary glands using fine needle aspiration has also been described [61], but there are no reports on the use of brush or exfoliative cytology. Salivary gland tumors of the palate may be amenable to sampling without fine needle aspiration technique because of the thin epithelium covering the palate and the greater likelihood that it will become ulcerated or traumatized, uncovering the subepithelial space. The cytology of these tumors on oral smear is similar to that in other sites, with a biphasic appearance showing an admixture of uniform epithelial cells with scanty, pale staining cytoplasm, and round to oval nuclei arranged in flat sheets, tubules, or papillary configurations, and spindle mesenchymal cells in a myxoid matrix that stains green-gray with Papanicolaou stain [62]. Figure 5.12a, b.

Peripheral Ameloblastoma

Peripheral ameloblastoma is a tumor of the oral cavity not involving bone but exhibiting microscopic features of ameloblastic differentiation. Most reported cases have occurred in the gingiva and may, on cytology, resemble basal cell carcinoma [63, 64].

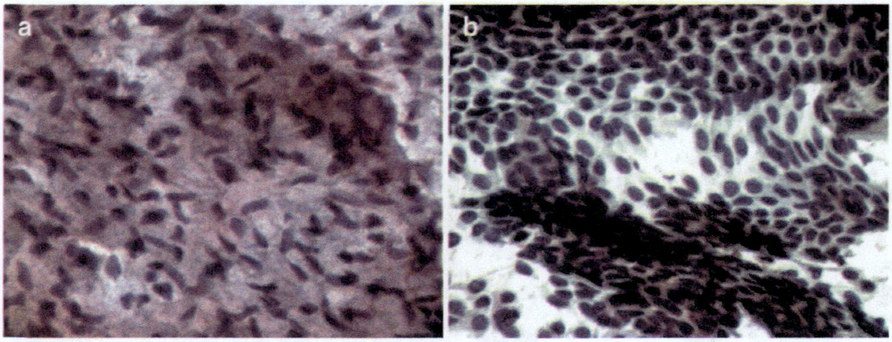

Fig. 5.12 Pleomorphic adenoma: (**a**) Tissue fragment showing spindle cells in myxoid matrix. (**b**) Sheets and tubules of uniform small cells with scanty cytoplasm

These may arise from remnants of the dental lamina within the gingiva or from the surface epithelium. Cytologically, they present with polarized tall columnar epithelial cells resembling the inner dental epithelium of the developing tooth follicle (ameloblasts) associated with a loose network of cells with elongated nuclei resembling the stellate reticulum of the enamel organ [63, 64]. Figure 5.13a, b.

Mucocele

The mucocele is one of the most common non-bony oral exophytic lesions [65]. It is believed to result from trauma or obstruction to a salivary gland excretory duct. The most common type (>90%), the extravasation cyst or mucus extravasation phenomenon, is a pseudocyst lined by granulation tissue formed in response to extravasated mucus. The less common retention cyst has a true epithelial lining. Clinically, these lesions present most commonly in the second to third decade of life, and appear as small, soft, translucent painless swellings which may be the normal mucosal color or blue. Locations include most commonly the lower lip, followed in frequency by the floor of the mouth and buccal mucosa [66, 67]. Brush biopsy smears will present with a mucoid background, benign appearing squamous cells, neutrophils, and abundant macrophages many with vacuolated cytoplasm corresponding to the muciphages seen in histologic sections [62, 66, 67]. Figure 5.14.

Peripheral Giant Cell Granuloma

Peripheral giant cell granuloma is a rare reactive exophytic lesion occurring on the gingiva and alveolar ridge, usually as a result of local irritating factors. It is also known as giant cell epulis, giant cell reparative granuloma, and osteoclastoma [68–70].

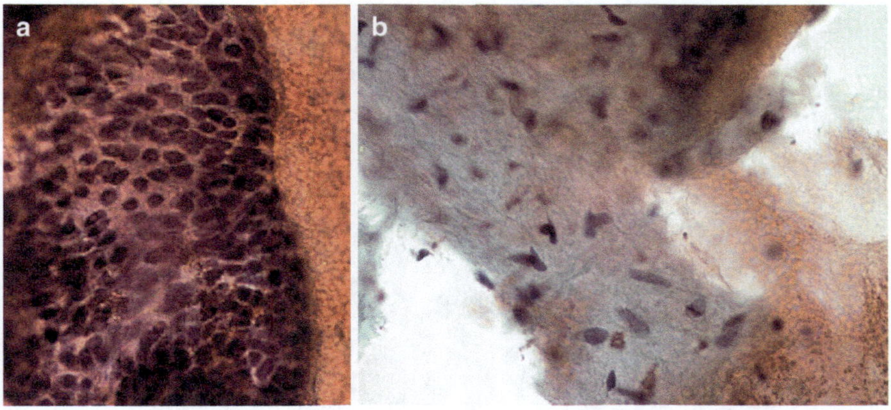

Fig. 5.13 Peripheral ameloblastoma: (**a**) Polarized columnar epithelial cells (ameloblasts). (**b**) Loose network of elongate nuclei that resembles stellate reticulum of the enamel organ

Histology will show young connective tissue cells and multinucleated giant cells, hemosiderin, hemorrhage, and inflammatory cells. Brush biopsy smears reveal a bloody background with variable numbers of inflammatory cells, scattered multinucleated giant cells, and scattered spindle cells. Figure 5.15.

Focal Fibrous Hyperplasia (Peripheral Fibroma and Traumatic Fibroma)

Focal fibrous hyperplasias, reactive lesions usually resulting from chronic trauma, are the most common non-bony exophytic oral lesions [65]. When present on the gingiva, they may be termed peripheral fibromas; when in other oral locations (most frequently the buccal mucosa, lateral tongue and lip), they may be called traumatic fibromas. The typical clinical presentation is of a raised, broad based, painless lesion that is paler than the surrounding mucosa [71]. Fibrous hyperplasias subjected to vigorous brush biopsy sampling or with surface ulceration may reveal benign squamous cells, some anucleate keratinocytes, and spindle cells in varying numbers. Connective tissue spindle cells may also appear in specimens from ulcerated lesions in the absence of fibrous hyperplasia [23]. In such situations, only rare cells will be present with background features consistent with ulceration. Figure 5.16a, b.

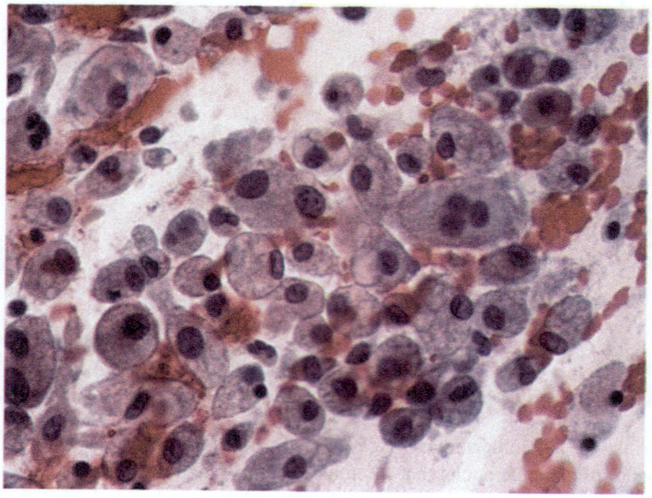

Fig. 5.14 Macrophages with vacuolated cytoplasm, blood, and scattered neutrophils from brush biopsy of mucocele

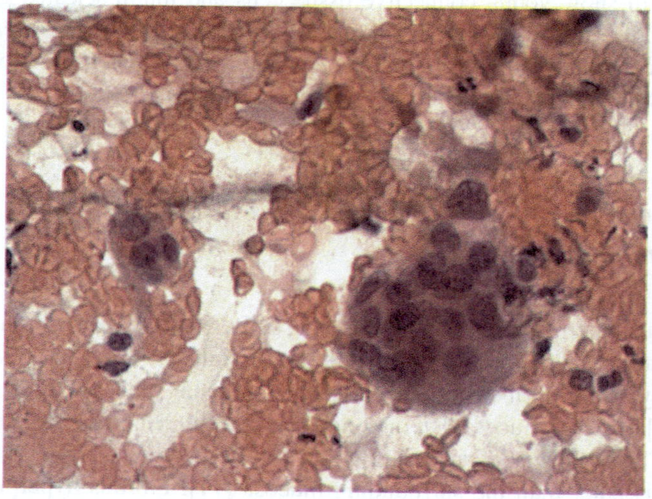

Fig. 5.15 Brush biopsy specimen from peripheral giant cell granuloma with multinucleated giant cell and inflammatory cells in a bloody background

Non-specific Inflammatory Changes

A variety of benign inflammatory conditions such as gingivitis, lichen planus, and traumatic, chronic, or apthous ulcers are red lesions or mixed red and white lesions which may undergo oral brush biopsy sampling if they are present with uncertain history and

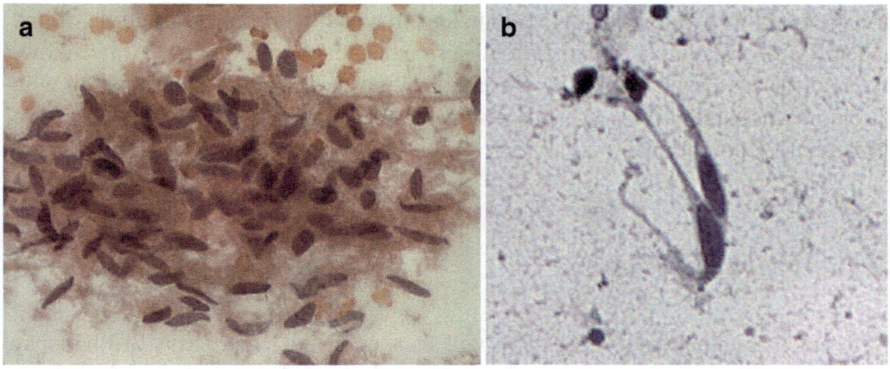

Fig. 5.16 Focal fibrous hyperplasia: (**a**) Tissue fragment of spindle cells in collagenous matrix from traumatic fibroma. (**b**) Rare spindle cells from subepithelium in brush biopsy sampling of ulcer

duration. The clinical concern over red or mixed color lesions is the result of the recognized significant association of erythroplakia with dysplasia and carcinoma [72].

Many benign inflammatory conditions will show non-specific changes even on histopathologic examination. Cytopathologic evaluation reveals varying combinations of features in the spectrum of changes characteristic of cell response to injury. Recognition of these benign cellular changes is important so as to clearly distinguish reactive atypias from atypia associated with premalignant or malignant change.

Cytoplasmic Features

Cell cytoplasm in reactive processes will show various degenerative changes including vacuolization, cytoplasmic extensions, and ill-defined cell borders [44]. Cytoplasm is opaque and staining with modified Pap may be biphasic (cyanophilic/eosinophilic). Notably absent are cells with transparent, refractile cytoplasm and crisp, clearly defined cell membranes.

Nuclear Features

Reactive nuclear features include varying combinations of binucleation or multinucleation and nuclear enlargement with hypochromia. Nuclear membranes may be indistinct. Chromatin is "powdery" or may appear blurred, especially in slightly air dried preparations. Alternatively, the nucleus may show prominent multiple, round nucleoli with vesicular chromatin. Small perinuclear halos are common. Anitschkow-like nuclear changes may also be present. Previously described in association with chronic apthous stomatitis [76], they may be seen nonspecifically in a variety of inflammatory conditions.

Tissue Fragment Features

Many reactive inflammatory conditions will show epithelial hyperplasia. Brush biopsy specimens will demonstrate tissue fragments—either with hyperplasia of uniform, regularly spaced basal cells, or of intermediate-sized cells with more abundant cytoplasm and reactive nuclear features as described above. Benign hyperkeratosis, parakeratosis and cytoplasmic granulosis may also be present. Anisonucleosis, individual cell necrosis, and significant nuclear crowding or irregular spacing should be absent.

Background Features

The smear background may contain neutrophils, red blood cells, and even fragments of fibrinopurulent exudate or granulation tissue but lacks necrotic cells or watery fluid. Abundant bacteria including numerous aggregates of Actinomyces sometimes admixed with cocci may be present, especially in cases clinically consistent with gingivitis (Fig. 5.17a–h).

Lichen Planus

Most of the lesions which have histologically proven to be lichen planus will show only non-specific inflammatory changes. The primary utility of brush biopsy sampling is as a useful adjunct to the periodic clinical assessment of lesions confirmed by histopathologic evaluation to be oral lichen planus. A small percentage of patients with oral lichen planus will ultimately develop squamous cell carcinoma, especially if the lichen planus is of the erosive subtype [73–75]. Cytology can play a role by identifying dysplastic or suspicious cells, prompting scalpel biopsy evaluation.

Two cytopathologic features are often present in smears from oral lichen planus which are not typically evident in other inflammatory conditions: a background inflammatory infiltrate which is predominantly lymphocytic, and tissue fragments showing both intraepithelial lymphocytes and occasional round homogeneous structures that look like the civatte or colloid bodies seen in histopathologic specimens [77] (Fig. 5.18a, b).

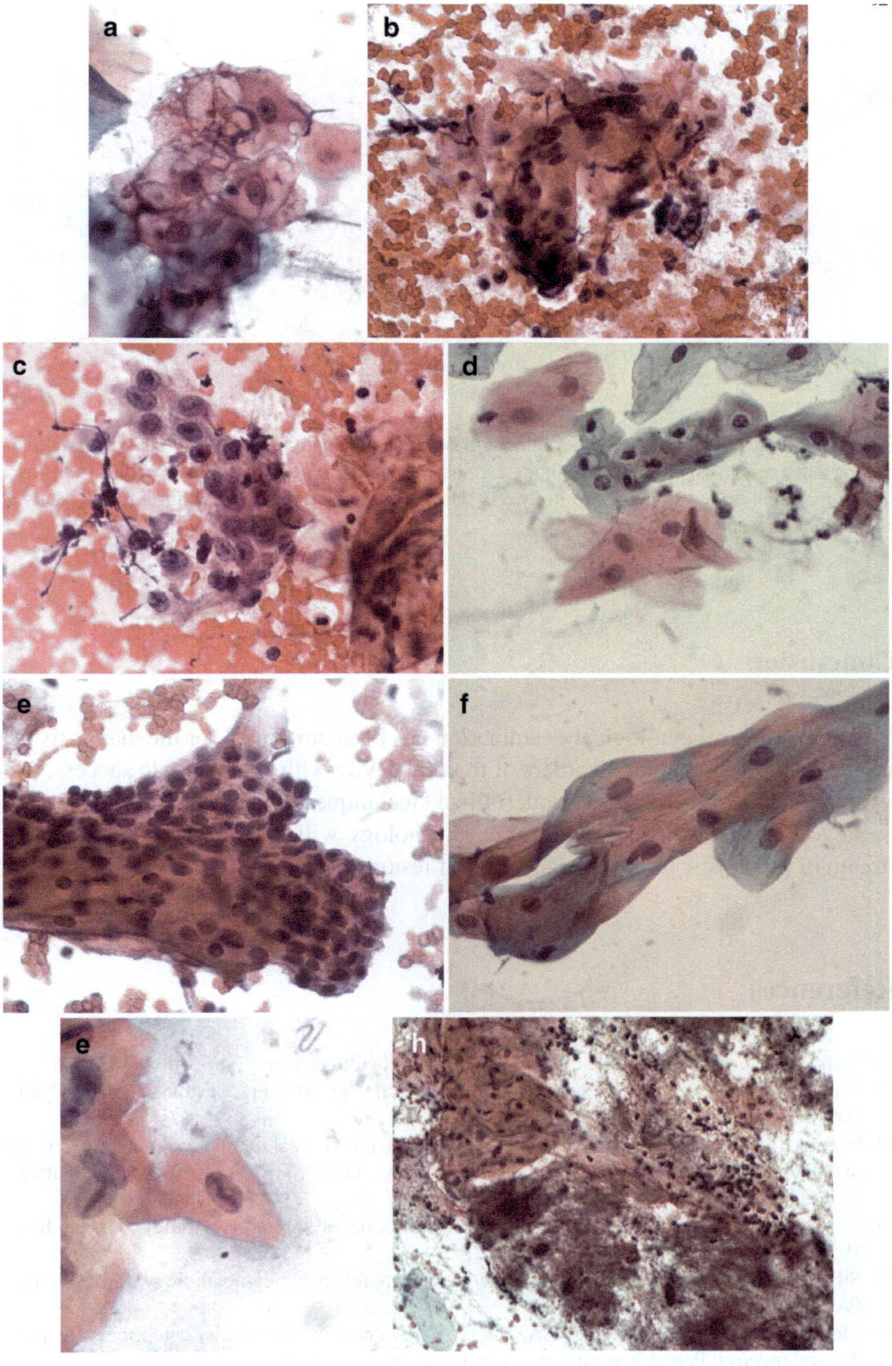

Fig. 5.17 Nonspecific inflammatory changes: (**a**) Cytoplasmic vacuolization. (**b**) Reactive multinucleation. (**c**) Tissue fragment showing reactive nuclei with enlargement, vesicular chromatin, and prominent nucleoli. (**d**) Small perinuclear halos. (**e**) Tissue fragment with basal cell hyperplasia. (**f**) Tissue fragment illustrating reactive features of nuclear enlargement, pale, "powdery" chromatin, and biphasic cytoplasmic staining. (**g**) Anitschkow-like nuclear changes. (**h**) Typical background with acute inflammatory infiltrate, blood, and many bacteria, predominately Actinomyces and cocci

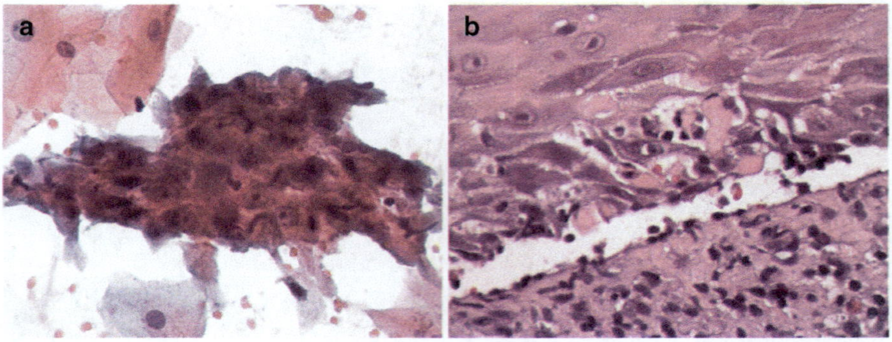

Fig. 5.18 Lichen planus: (**a**) Tissue fragment from brush biopsy of lichen planus showing reactive nuclear changes, intraepithelial lymphocytes, and intraepithelial eosinophilic structure (*top, just right of center*) suggesting civatte body. (**b**) Histopathology section showing similar reactive nuclear features and civatte bodies

Conclusion

In conclusion, oral cytological examination has been employed for the diagnosis of a wide plethora of benign disorders of the oral cavity with considerable success. As awareness about this relatively underutilized technique spreads and novel technologies evolve, it is estimated that oral cytopathology will soon be part of the mainstream of diagnostic tools for evaluation of lesions of the oral cavity.

References

1. Selbach CJ, vonHamm E. The clinical value of oral cytology. Acta Cytol. 1963;7:337–45.
2. Sandler HC. Detection of early cancer of mouth by exfoliative cytology. Acta Cytol. 1961;5:191–4.
3. Folsom TC, White CP, Bromer L, Canby HF, Garrington G. Oral exfoliative study. Review of the literature and report of a three-year study. Oral Surg Oral Med Oral Pathol. 1972;33(1):61–74.
4. Silverman S, Becks H, Farber SM. Diagnostic value of intraoral cytology. J Dent Res. 1958;37:195–205.
5. Silverman S. Oral cavity. In: Bibbo M, editor. Comprehensive cytopathology. Philadelphia, PA: WB Saunders; 1991. p. 399–408.
6. Medack H, Burlakow P, McGrew EA, Tiecke R. The cytology of vesicular conditions affecting the oral mucosa: Pemphigus vulgaris. Acta Cytol. 1970;14:11–21.
7. Mehrotra R. The role of cytology in oral lesions: a review of recent improvements. Diag Cytopathol. 2012;40:73–83.
8. Mehrotra R, Hullmann M, Smeets R, Reichert TE, Driemel O. Oral cytology revisited. J Oral Pathol Med. 2009;38(2):161–6.

9. Sciubba JJ. Improving detection of precancerous and cancerous oral lesions. Computer-assisted analysis of the oral brush biopsy. U.S. Collaborative OralCDx Study Group. J Am Dent Assoc. 1999;130(10):1445–57.
10. Scheifele C, Schmidt-Westhausen AM, Dietrich T, Reichart PA. The sensitivity and specificity of the OralCDx technique: evaluation of 103 cases. Oral Oncol. 2004;40(8):824–8.
11. Patton LL, Epstein JB, Kerr AR. Adjunctive techniques for oral cancer examination and lesion diagnosis: a systematic review of the literature. J Am Dent Assoc. 2008;139(7):896–905.
12. Lingen MW, Kalmar JR, Karrison T, Speight PM. Critical evaluation of diagnostic aids for the detection of oral cancer. Oral Oncol. 2008;44(1):10–22.
13. Mehrotra R, et al. The efficacy of oral brush biopsy with computer-assisted analysis in identifying precancerous and cancerous lesions. Head Neck Oncol. 2011;3:39. doi:10.1186/1758-3284-3-39.
14. Burzynski NJ, Firriolo FJ, Butters JM, Sorrell CL. Evaluation of oral cancer screening. J Cancer Educ. 1997;12(2):95–9.
15. Reboiras-López MD, Pérez-Sayáns M, Somoza-Martín JM, Gayoso-Diz P, Barros-Angueira F, Gándara-Rey JM, García-García A. Comparison of the Cytobrush®, dermatological curette and oral CDx® brush test as methods for obtaining samples of RNA for molecular analysis of oral cytology. Cytopathology. 2011. doi: 10.1111/j.1365-2303.2011.00860.x.
16. Pérez-Sayánsm M, Somoza-Martín JM, Barros-Angueira F, Reboiras-López MD, Gándara-Vila P, Gándara Rey JM, García-García A. Exfoliative cytology for diagnosing oral cancer. Biotech Histochem. 2010;85(3):177–87.
17. Ogden GR, Cowpe JG, Wright AJ. Oral exfoliative cytology: review of methods of assessment. J Oral Pathol Med. 1997;26(5):201–5.
18. Regezi JA, Sciubba JJ, Jordan RCK. White lesions. In: Regezi JA, Sciubba JJ, Jordan RCK, editors. Oral pathology: clinical pathologic correlations. 5th ed. St Louis, MO: Saunders Elsevier; 2008. p. 73–106.
19. Pindborg JJ, Jolst O, Renstrup G, Roed-Petersen B. Studies in oral leukoplakia: a preliminary report on the period prevalence of malignant transformation in leukoplakia based on a follow-up study of 248 patients. J Am Dent Assoc. 1968;76:767–71.
20. Waldron CA, Shafer WG. Leukoplakia revisited: aclinicopathologic study of 3256 oral leukoplakias. Cancer. 1975;36(4):1386–92.
21. Bouquot JE. Common oral lesions found during a mass screening examination. J Am Dent Assoc. 1986;112(1):50–7.
22. Oral CDx Laboratories, Case Database query. Unpublished.
23. Medak H, McGrew EA, Brulakow P, Tiecke RW. Atlas of oral cytology. US department of Health Education and Welfare Publication No 1949. 1970.
24. Bouquot JE, Gorlin RJ. Leukoplakia, lichen planus, and other oral keratoses in 23,616 white Americans over the age of 35 years. Oral Surg Oral Med Oral Pathol. 1986;61:373–81.
25. Napier SS, Speight PM. Natural history of potentially malignant oral lesions and conditions: an overview of the literature. J Oral Pathol Med. 2008;37(1):1–10.
26. Gonsalves WC, Chi AC, Neville BW. Common oral lesions: part I superficial mucosal lesions. Am Fam Physician. 2007;75:501–7.
27. Reamy BV, Derby R, Bunt CW. Common tongue conditions in primary care. Am Fam Physician. 2010;81(5):627–34.
28. Daniels TE, Hansen LS, Greenspan JS, Grady DG, Hauck WW, Greene JC, Ernster VL. Histopathology of smokeless tobacco lesions in professional baseball players. Associations with different types of tobacco. Oral Surg Oral Med Oral Pathol. 1992;73(6):720–5.
29. Greer RO. Oral manifestations of smokeless tobacco use. Otolaryngol Clin North Am. 2011;44(1):31–56.
30. Taybos G. Oral changes associated with tobacco use. Am J Med Sci. 2003;326(4):179–82.
31. Roberts DM. Comparative cytology of the oral cavities of snuff users. Acta Cytol. 1997;41(4):1008–14.
32. Patil R, Nayak S, Munshi M, Bobhate S. Scrape cytology in rare case of hairy tongue. J Cytol. 2009;26(2):91–3.
33. Nisa L, Giger R. Black hairy tongue. Am J Med. 2011;124(9):816–7.

34. Reginald A, Sivapathasundharam B. Oral hairy leukoplakia: an exfoliative cytology study. Contemp Clin Dent. 2010;1(1):10–3.
35. Migliorati CA, Jones AC, Baughman PA. Use of exfoliative cytology in the diagnosis or oral hairy leukoplakia. Oral Surg Oral Med Oral Pathol. 1993;76(6):704–10.
36. Gelardi M, Tomaiuolo M, Cassano M, Besozzi G, Fiorella ML, Calvario A, Castellano MA, Cassano P. Epstein-barr virus induced cellular changes in nasal mucosa. Virol J. 2006;3:6. doi:10.1186/1743-422X-3-6.
37. Walling DM, Flaitz CM, Adler-Storthz K, Nichiols CM. A non-invasive technique for studying oral epithelial Epstein Barr infection and disease. Oral Oncol. 2003;39(5):436–44.
38. Shulman JD, Beach MM, Rivera-Hidalgo F. The prevalence of oral mucosal lesions in U.S. adults: data from the Third National Health and Nutrition Examination Survey, 1988–1994. JAMA. 2004;135(9):1279–86.
39. Akpan A, Morgan R. Oral candidiasis. Postgrad Med J. 2002;78:455–9.
40. Loss R, Sandrin R, França BHS, de Azevedo-Alanis LR, Grégio AMT, Machado MÂN, Lima AAS. Cytological analysis of the epithelial cells in patients with oral candidiasis. Mycoses. 2011;54:e130–5. doi:10.1111/j.1439-0507.2009.01857.x.
41. Buchner A, Hansen LS. Lymphoepithelial cysts of the oral mucosa. Oral Surg Oral Med Oral Pathol. 1980;50:441–9.
42. Chaudhry AP. A clinicopathologic study of intraoral lymphoepithelial cysts. J Oral Med. 1984;39:79–84.
43. Nonaka CF, Henriques AC, de Matos FR, de Souza LB, Pinto LP. Nonodontogenic cysts of the oral and maxillofacial region: demographic profile in a Brazilian population over a 40-year period. Eur Arch Otorhinolaryngol. 2011;268(6):917–22.
44. Ramzy I. Gynecologic infections. In: Ramzy I, editor. Clinical cytopathology & aspiration biopsy: fundamental principles and practice. Norwalk, CT: Appleton & Lange; 1990. p. 221–2.
45. Gupta LK, Singhi MK. Tzanck smear: a useful diagnostic tool. Indian J Dermatol Venerol Leprol. 2005;71:295–9.
46. Chauvin PJ, Ajar AH. Acute herpetic gingivostomatitis in adults: a review of 13 cases including diagnosis and management. J Can Dent Assoc. 2002;68(4):247–51.
47. Brown RS, Eiland D. Palatal lesions in an otherwise healthy patient. J Am Dent Assoc. 2010;141(4):429–32.
48. Kobayashi TK, Ueda M, Nishino T, et al. Brush cytology of Herpes simplex virus infection in oral mucosa. Use of the Thin Prep processor. Diagn Cytopathol. 1998;18:71–5.
49. Epithelial lesions of the oral cavity, larynx, trachea, nasopharynx, and paranasal sinuses. In: Koss LG, Melamed MR, editors. Koss' diagnostic cytology and it's histopathologic bases, 5th ed. Philadelphia, PA: Lippincott Williams &Wilkins; 2006. p. 713–37.
50. Benign disorders of the uterine cervix and vagina. In: Koss LG, Melamed MR, editors. Koss' diagnostic cytology and it's histopathologic bases, 5th ed. Philadelphia, PA: Lippincott Williams &Wilkins; 2006. p. 241–81.
51. McKenzie CD, Gobrtt JP. Diagnosis and treatment of profacial herpes zoster:report of cases. J Am Dent Assoc. 1990;120(6):679–81.
52. Robinson NA, Yoe JF, Lee YS, Aw DCW. Oral pemphigus vulgaris: a case report and literature update. Ann Acad Med Singapore. 2004;33(Suppl):63s–8.
53. Scully C, Mignogna M. Oral mucosal disease: pemphigus. Br J Oral Maxillofac Surg. 2008;46(4):272–7.
54. Kobayashi TK, Kaneko C, Sugishima S, Kusukawa J, Kameyama T. Scrape cytology of oral pemphigus: report of a case with immunocytochemistry and light, scanning electron, and transmission electron microscopy. Acta Cytol. 1999;43(2):289–94.
55. Regezi JA, Sciubba JJ, Jordan RCK. Pigmented lesions. In: Regezi JA, Sciubba JJ, Jordan RCK, editors. Oral pathology: clinical pathologic correlations. 5th ed. St Louis, MO: Saunders Elsevier; 2008. p. 127–39.
56. Buchner A, Merrell PW, Carpenter WM. Relative frequency of solitary melanocytic lesions of the oral mucosa. J Oral Pathol Med. 2004;33(9):550–7.

57. Page LR, Corio RL, Crawford Giansanti JS, Weathers DR. The oral melanotic macule. Oral Surg Oral Med Oral Pathol. 1977; 44(2): 219–26.
58. Everson JW, Cawson RA. Tumors of the minor (oropharyngeal) salivary gland. A demographic study of 336 cases. J Oral Pathol. 1985;14:500–9.
59. Waldron CA, el-Mofty SK, Gnepp DR. Tumors of the intraoral minor salivary glands: a demographic and histologic study of 426 cases. Oral Surg Oral Med Oral Pathol. 1988;66(3):323–33.
60. Dhanuthai K, Sappayatosok K, Kongin K. Pleomorphic adenoma of the palate in a child: a case report. Med Oral Pathol Oral Cir Buccal. 2009;14(2):E73–5.
61. Shah SB, Singe MI, Liberman E, Ljung BM. Transmucosal fine needle aspiration diagnosis of intraoral and intrapharyngeal lesions. Laryngoscope. 1999;109:1232–7.
62. Elhosseiny A. Salivary glands. In: Koss LG, Melamed MR, editors. Koss' diagnostic cytology and it's histopathologic bases. 5th ed. Philadelphia, PA: Lippincott Williams &Wilkins; 2006. p. 1229–61.
63. Gardner DG. Peripheral ameloblastoma: a study of 21 cases, including 5 reported as basal cell carcinoma of the gingiva. Cancer. 1977;39:1625–33.
64. LeCorn DW, Bhattacharyya I, Vertucci FJ. Peripheral ameloblastoma: a case report and review of the literature. J Endod. 2006;32(2):152–4.
65. Bouquot JE, Gundlach KK. Oral exophytic lesions in 23,616 white Americans over 35 years of age. Oral Surg Oral Med Oral Pathol. 1986; 62(3).
66. Oliveira DT, Consolaro A, Freitas FJ. Histopathological spectrum of 112 cases of mucocele. Braz Dent J. 1993;4(1):29–36.
67. Hayashida AM, Zerbinatti DCZ, Balducci I, Cabral LAG, Almeida JD. Mucus extravasation and retention phenomena: a 24 year study. BMC Oral Health. 2010;10:15. doi:10.1186/1472-6831-10-15.
68. Shadman N, Ebrahimi SF, Jafari S, Eslami M. Peripheral giant cell granuloma: a review of 123 cases. Dent Res J (Isfahan). 2009;6(1):47–50.
69. Chaparro-Avendano AV, Berini-Aytes L, Gay-Escoda C. Peripheral giant cell granuloma: a report of five case and review of the literature. Med Oral Pathol Oral Ar Bucal. 2005;10(1):53–7. 48–52.
70. Giansanti JS, Waldron CA. Peripheral giant cell granuloma, review of 720 cases. J Oral Surg. 1969;27:787–91.
71. Regezi JA, Sciubba JJ, Jordan RCK. Connective tissue lesions. In: Regezi JA, Sciubba JJ, Jordan RCK, editors. Oral pathology: clinical pathologic correlations. 5th ed. St Louis, MO: Saunders Elsevier; 2008. p. 155–77.
72. Reichart PA, Philllipsen HP. Oral erythroplakia – a review. Oral Oncol. 2005;41:551–61.
73. Abbate G, Foscolo AM, Gallotti M, Lancella A, Mingo F. Neoplastic transformation of oral lichen: case report and review of the literature. Acta Otorhinolaryngol Ital. 2006;26(1):47–51.
74. Barnard NA, Scully C, Everson JW, Cunningham S, Proter SR. Oral cancer development in patients with oral lichen planus. J Oral Pathol Med. 1993;22(9):421–4.
75. Chainani-Wu N, Silverman S, Lozada-Nur F, Mayer P, Watson JJ. Oral lichen planus: patient profile, disease progression and treatment responses. J Am Dent Assoc. 2001;132(7):901–9.
76. Wood TA, De Witt SH, Chu EW, Rabson AS, Graykowski EA. Anitschkow nuclear changes observed in oral smears. Acta Cytol. 1975;19(5):434–7.
77. Sugerman PB, Savage NW, Walsh LJ, Zhao ZZ, Zhou XJ, Khan A, Seymour GJ, Bigby M. The pathogenesis of oral lichen planus. Crit Rev Oral Biol Med. 2002;13(4):350–65.

Chapter 6
The Development of a Novel Oral Cytologic Grading System

Amir Afrogheh, Jos Hille, and Ravi Mehrotra

Cervical cytology gained popularity with the publications of Papanicolaou and Traut, who demonstrated the diagnostic value of exfoliative cytology in the detection of carcinoma of the uterine cervix [1]. A variety of classification systems for reporting cervical cytology have been adopted since. In the "Papanicolaou" (Pap) classification, a specific "class" provided a level of concern about the presence of cancer cells. For example, class I smears contained benign cells and class V smears contained cells definitively diagnostic of malignancy.

The Pap classification system gradually became outdated as it had many variations and failed to keep abreast with the recent scientific advances in cervical carcinogenesis and precursor lesions [2]. Reagan encouraged the use of the term dysplasia for precancerous lesions, and dysplastic lesions were then subdivided by degree of abnormality and cell type, severe keratinizing dysplasia being an example [3, 4]. Richart introduced the term "Cervical Intraepithelial Neoplasia" (CIN) in 1967 to promote the idea of a continuum of precursor lesions [5].

The use of multiple classification systems for reporting results of cervical cytology soon caused widespread confusion among many laboratories and clinicians culminating in the development of a standard grading method. In 1988, the Bethesda system was developed to provide a uniform scheme for reporting cervical cytology, through a workshop convened by the National Cancer Institute (NCI) [2]. Subsequently, two additional workshops were held in 1999 and 2001 to address the inherent deficiencies of the new system and the role of evolving technologies and scientific advances in reporting [6, 7]. The 2001 Bethesda System received many

A. Afrogheh • J. Hille (✉)
TBH Laboratories, Oral & Maxillofacial Pathology, National Health Laboratory Service, University of the Western Cape, Cape Town, South Africa
e-mail: jhille@sun.ac.za

R. Mehrotra
Institute of Cytology and Preventive Oncology (ICPO), I-7, Sector - 39, Noida - 201301, Uttar Pradesh, India
e-mail: rm8509@gmail.com

R. Mehrotra (ed.), *Oral Cytology: A Concise Guide*, DOI 10.1007/978-1-4614-5221-8_6,

inputs from cytologists and cytotechnologists and was attended by more than 400 participants, preceded by internet discussion groups [7].

While the Bethesda classification method represents one of the great success stories in cervical cytology, there has been little appetite for the adoption of a universal grading for oral cytology. This could be explained by the general lack of interest in oral cytology, which is due to a high percentage of false negative diagnoses [8, 9], attributed to great variation in technical quality and cellularity of oral smears as well as the use of inadequate sampling procedures. The lack of a standardized method for reporting oral cytology adversely affects proper management of patients with oral lesions.

Many investigators have used or continue to use a three-tiered oral cytologic grading system on adequate samples [10–12], whilst others have failed to provide one [13–17]. In a study performed in 1983 to evaluate the role of fine needle aspiration (FNA) in squamous cell carcinomas of the head and neck, Feldman et al. reported 229 FNAs, 42 of which were from the oral region [10]. The FNA results were reported in one of four categories: unsatisfactory, negative, suspicious, or positive for malignancy. Similar criteria were used by Scher et al. in evaluating FNAs from the oral cavity, oropharynx and nasopharynx [11]. In this study, suspicious FNA specimens were proven to be malignant in 100% of the cases that underwent subsequent biopsy.

The brush biopsy (CDx Laboratories, Suffern, NY, USA) was introduced in 1999 as a potential oral cancer case-finding device. In a prospective multicenter study to determine the sensitivity and specificity of oral brush biopsy (OralCDx®) for detection of pre-cancerous and cancerous lesions of the oral mucosa, Sciubba et al. reported results as positive, atypical or negative [12].

Currently, most available oral diagnostic tissue tests are expensive, time-consuming, invasive and not within easy reach of the vast majority of the world population which needs these investigations the most. These diagnostic procedures also require training and present logistical issues, e.g. infection control, transport of samples, turnaround times, communication of results and patient travel for recall. Though these issues may not present too many constraints to patients and clinicians with access to well-equipped and easily accessible healthcare systems, there is a pressing requirement to develop simpler, inexpensive and minimally invasive devices/methodologies which enable the diagnosis of clinically significant oral lesions with a high degree of accuracy. This need is all the more evident in rural and economically disadvantaged, medically underserved areas. The presently existing oral cytology techniques are largely experimental and are undergoing extensive testing.

For now, the conventional Pap smear for cervical smears provides better diagnostic information through its more elaborate Bethesda grading system than the OralCDx® for oral smears. The emergence of Liquid-Based Cytology (LBC) in recent years with dramatic improvements in technical quality and cellularity of the cytology specimens [18] has provoked a new interest in oral cytology. This inspired the authors to conduct a recent study [19] using an economical liquid-based preparatory method (Shandon PapSpin™) and propose an oral cytologic grading method analogous to the Bethesda System for reporting cervical cytology (Table 6.1).

Table 6.1 Oral/oropharyngeal cytologic grading system

Grading system
Specimen adequacy
Adequate for evaluation (note the presence of basal/parabasal cells)
Inadequate for evaluation (specify reason, e.g. obscuring elements, unlabelled or broken slides)
General categorization
A: Normal
B: Reactive[a]
C: Atypical-probably reactive/low grade including low grade squamous intraepithelial lesion (LSIL)
D: Atypical-Probably high grade
E: High grade squamous intraepithelial lesion
F: Invasive squamous cell carcinoma
G: Other neoplasms: Specify

[a]The reactive category includes hyperkeratosis, inflammatory, infective, repair & chemo/radiation changes

The preservation of the traditional cytomorphologic criteria rendered by the PapSpin™ method allows standardization through both conventional and liquid-based cytologic techniques. Using this classification, the terminology for reporting results obtained by oral cytology examination is discussed.

Adequacy Criteria

The 2001 Bethesda guidelines for reporting cervical cytology [7] consider a conventional smear as adequately cellular, if the smear has an estimated minimum of at least 8,000–12,000 well preserved (not obscured by blood or inflammation) squamous cells. Conventional smears with more than 75% of the squamous cells obscured by blood or inflammation are designated as unsatisfactory for evaluation. Since liquid-based preparations (LBPs) have more random sampling of cell constituents, a lower minimum cellularity of 5,000 well preserved squamous cells is required.

Reference images are provided for the estimation of conventional smear cellularity; laboratories are not to count individual cells [20]. Cell numbers on LBPs are reproducibly evaluated by estimates of representative fields. Kujan et al. in 2006 reinforced the method to draw a line across the center of each preparation and to evaluate ten discontinuous fields across the middle diameter of each preparation using the 40× objective lens. Only well-visualized squamous cells are counted. Large groups containing more than five squamous cells are counted on only one plane of focus. The average cell count from the ten fields (40×) is measured. An average of at least 7 cells/field is required in order to achieve the minimum of 5,000 cells/preparation [14].

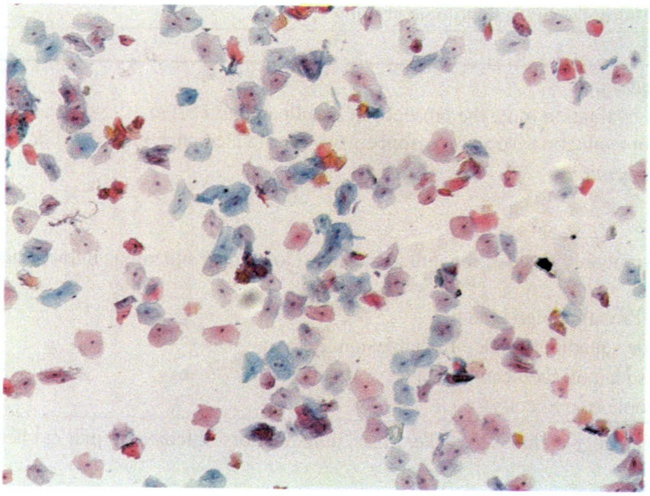

Fig. 6.1 LBC (PapSpin). An adequate oral sample. Approximately 60% of the diameter of the preparation (5 mm circle) is covered by cellular material (Pap stain, ×100)

While the Bethesda System provides a set of numeric criteria for minimal squamous cellularity of adequate cervical cytology specimens, such criteria are not well defined for oral cytology specimens. Conventional oral smears are generally more hypocellular than cervical smears and for this reason some investigators consider smears with at least 30 well preserved intermediate or parabasal cells (not obscured by blood, exudate or necrosis) as adequately cellular for evaluation [15], while others have failed to describe the criteria used [13, 16, 17] or have simply adhered to the adequacy criteria proposed by the Bethesda System [14]. In a study of normal oral mucosa using the SurePath™ LBC method and applying the Bethesda adequacy criteria, only two of the 150 (1.3%) specimens evaluated were considered inadequate, however, only 6 of the 150 slides studied contained basal cells.

In general, a suitable oral cytologic specimen should contain a representative sample of superficial, intermediate and parabasal/basal cells; and it is therefore important to assess the presence of the latter cells within specimens of adequate squamous cellularity (Table 6.1). The proper application of the Transepithelial Brush Biopsy Technique (TBBT) [12, 19, 21, 22] results in a significantly improved harvest of basal and parabasal cells. With TBBT, the brush is firmly applied to the lesion and rotated a number of times until pin point (punctuate) bleeding is provoked. This ensures a full thickness epithelial sampling via a minimally invasive procedure and provides the oral pathologist with a more representative cytologic specimen of the brushed mucosal epithelium.

In our recent study using the PapSpin™ LBC technique [19], a specimen was considered inadequate if less than 30% of the diameter of the circle of cells (5 mm) was covered by cellular material (Fig. 6.1). Although we deem this a simple and time saving adequacy criterion for LBPs, it may prove difficult for other non-calibrated examiners to reproducibly apply this principle. It is therefore prudent

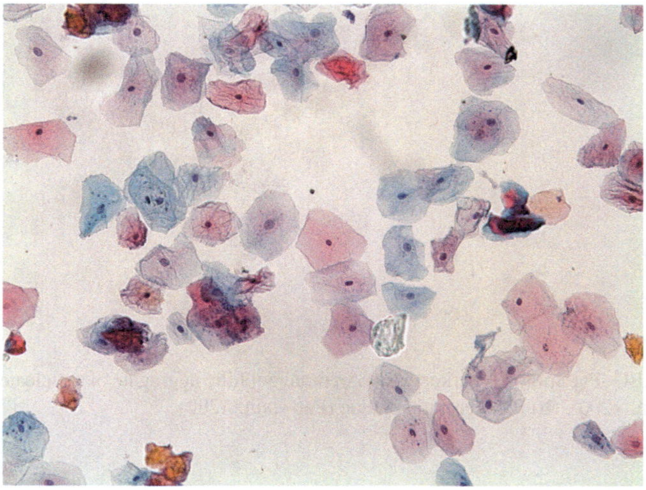

Fig. 6.2 LBC (PapSpin). Even distribution of oral superficial and intermediate cells (Pap stain, ×400)

to state that future prospective studies will have to confirm this proposed standard or suggest alternative assessment criteria to determine the minimum squamous cellularity of oral cytologic specimens. Until such time, it is recommended to use the adequacy criteria proposed by the 2001 Bethesda system.

General Diagnostic Categorization

A: Normal

The oral stratified squamous epithelium consists of several layers. The basal layer appears as a single, well organized row of darkly staining cells that rest on a basement membrane. These cells together with the immediately superficial parabasal cells (Fig. 6.4a) are responsible for the continuous renewal of the oral epithelium. As the cells progressively migrate toward the surface, they acquire increased cytoplasm, the nature of which is eosinophilic due to increased cytokeratin protein deposition. Thus, the most mature cells in the upper layers of the epithelium have extremely small pyknotic nuclei and abundant eosinophilic cytoplasm and are known as superficial cells (Fig. 6.2).

The intermediate cells are characterized by pale grooved nuclei, the open chromatin of which may occasionally reveal a small chromocenter (Fig. 6.2). The cytoplasm of intermediate cells may contain abundant glycogen particles and appear clear in Pap-stained preparations.

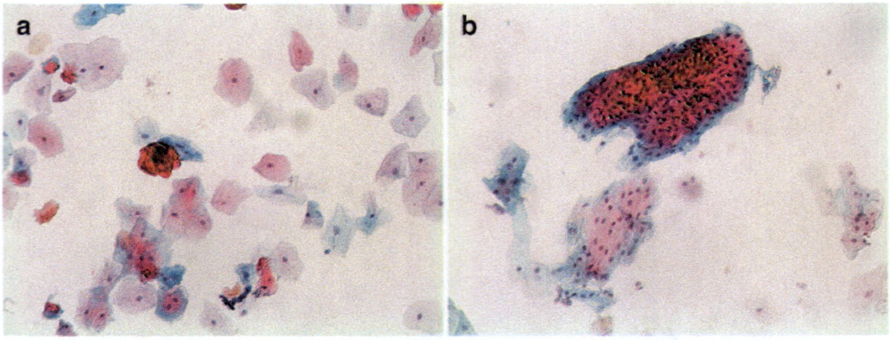

Fig. 6.3 (**a**) LBC (PapSpin). Hyperkeratosis. An orangeophilic aggregate of anucleated superficial cells (Pap stain, ×200). (**b**) Parakeratotic plaque (Pap stain, ×200)

It is not surprising to see basal and parabasal cells in smears/preparations from atrophic oral epithelia. The basal/parabasal cells have scanty basophilic (protein poor) cytoplasm and nuclei that are larger than those of intermediate cells. This results in a high nuclear/cytoplasmic ratio. However, their nuclear membrane is smooth and regular and the chromatin is pale and delicate (Fig. 6.4a). In keratinized masticatory mucosa (hard plate and gingiva), anucleated keratotic superficial cells may be seen (orthokeratosis) or parakeratotic cells/plaques (parakeratosis—Fig. 6.3a, b) and these should be regarded as normal. However, the finding of hyperkeratotic cells derived from a white mucosal lesion in the presence of normal basal cells should be included in the reactive category. The parakeratotic cells generally have orangeophilic cytoplasm and small pyknotic nuclei, in which no residual chromatin structure is identified. Abnormally configured keratotic cells should be viewed with caution as they may herald an underlying dysplastic/malignant process.

B: Reactive

Oral squamous cells undergo reactive cytological alterations in the presence of a number of conditions. For this reason the reactive category is further subcategorized into infectious, inflammatory, repair and chemo-/radiotherapy induced changes.

(1) Inflammation/Infective

In the presence of an inflammatory/infective process, the smear/preparation often contains an infiltrate of acute inflammatory cells with predominance of neutrophils (except

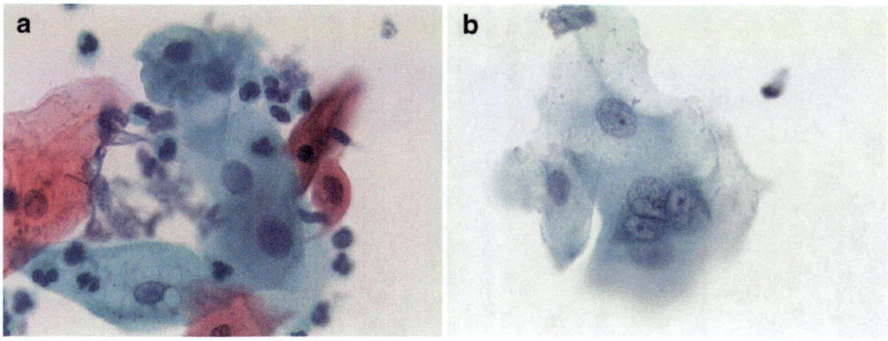

Fig. 6.4 (**a**) LBC (PapSpin). Reactive (inflammatory)-an aphthous ulcer. In addition to the normal intermediate cells (*left*), this image shows cells (*center*) with a generous body of mature cytoplasm and mild nuclear enlargement with an attendant slight increase in N:C ratio. Hyperchromasia is not evident and the nuclear outlines are smooth. A basal/parabasal cell is seen on the right. The cell shows a marked increase in N:C ratio, resembling a high grade squamous intraepithelial lesion, but hyperchromasia is minimal and the nuclear outline is smooth (Pap stain, ×1,000). (**b**) Reactive. Multinucleated cell with abundant cytoplasm. The nuclei are normochromatic and the nuclear outlines are smooth. The chromatin is finely granular and evenly distributed. Small nucleoli are noted, suggesting a reactive process (Pap stain, ×1,000)

in automated liquid-based preparations). Eosinophils are rarely seen in fixed oral smears/preparations, since the distinctive red granules are lost. A dense inflammatory infiltrate may partially or fully obscure oral squamous epithelial cells in conventional oral smears. This together with the hypocellular nature of the oral smears in general may result in inadequate specimens.

The inflammatory infiltrate is markedly reduced in liquid based preparations based on cytocentrifugation (e.g. PapSpin™) and is almost non-existent in automated liquid-based preparations, e.g. Thin Prep™ (Cytec Corporation, Boxborough, MA). Nevertheless, given the large number of inflammatory/infective conditions encountered in the oral region, the presence of these cells is desirable, allowing a precise cytologic diagnosis to be made.

The cells in these subcategories often have a generous body of cytoplasm and demonstrate mild nuclear enlargement with an attendant slight increase in nuclear to cytoplasmic (N:C) ratio (Fig. 6.4a). Cells with hyperchromatic nuclei are not seen, however, small perinuclear halos, cytoplasmic vacuolation (Fig. 6.4a), and bi-/multinucleated cells (Fig. 6.4b) may be seen as part of the reactive changes. *Candida* spp. cause the most common fungal infection of oral mucosa and are detected in oral smears/preparations as budding yeasts and pseudohyphae (Fig. 6.5a). The finding of granulomas in oral cytologic smears/preparations underlines the importance of oral cytology as a rapid and reliable test for diagnosing oral granulomatous conditions, e.g. tuberculosis and histoplasmosis (Fig. 6.5b, c).

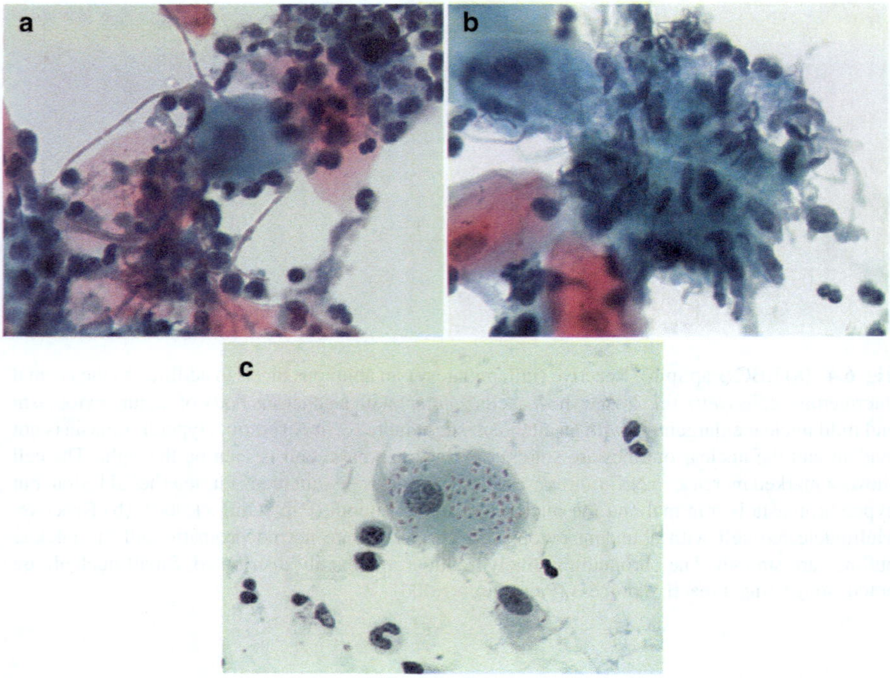

Fig. 6.5 (**a**) LBC (PapSpin). Reactive (infective)—this image shows pseudohyphae of *Candida* spp. with a marked acute inflammatory cell response. The cell in the center displays reactive cellular changes, mild nuclear enlargement with an attendant increase in N:C ratio. However, nuclear hyperchromasia is not present and the nuclear outline is smooth. (**b**) Granuloma from an irregular ulcer with rolled/heaped up margins on the hard palate, clinically thought to be a squamous cell carcinoma. The image shows a cluster of epithelioid cells arranged in a syncytial fashion. The cells have oval to slightly bent nuclei and delicate cytoplasm (Pap stain, ×1,000). (**c**) Histoplasmosis. In addition to granulomas, a macrophage is seen containing numerous small intracellular round to oval bodies, 1–5 μm yeast cells, surrounded by a small light halo (Pap stain, ×1,000)

(2) Repair

The oral cavity is a common site where a number of benign ulcerative conditions occur. These include aphthous ulcers, vesiculo-bullous diseases and traumatic ulcers, all of which are characterized by episodes of ulceration and regeneration (repair). Most cytologic examples of repair are characterized by cells arranged in cohesive flat streaming sheets that are often associated with inflammatory cells.

The cells demonstrate enlarged but pale nuclei, with even nuclear contours and prominent nucleoli (Fig. 6.6). This cytomorphology may resemble that of a squamous cell carcinoma, however, no single cells with similar cytomorphology are identified in repair which is a clue to the correct cytologic diagnosis.

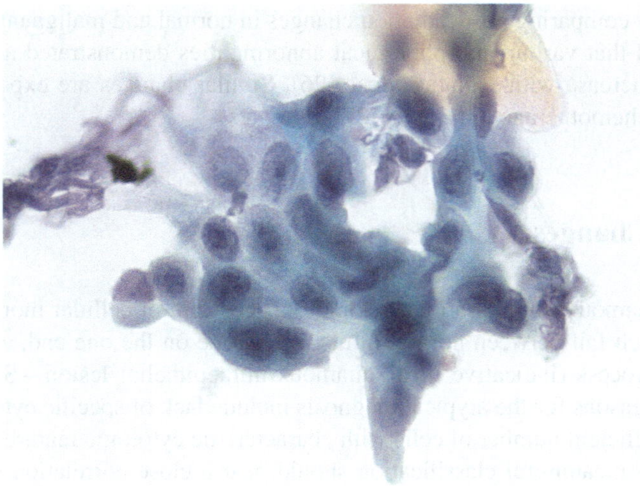

Fig. 6.6 LBC (PapSpin). Healing erosive lesion on the palate in a patient with oral mucous membrane pemphigoid. The cells are arranged in a flat streaming sheet. The nuclei are enlarged and show smooth to slightly irregular nuclear outlines and single prominent nucleoli. Mild hyperchromasia is seen although chromatin structure and distribution remains finely granular. No single cells with similar cytomorphology were identified, a key feature to correct diagnosis (Pap stain, ×1,000)

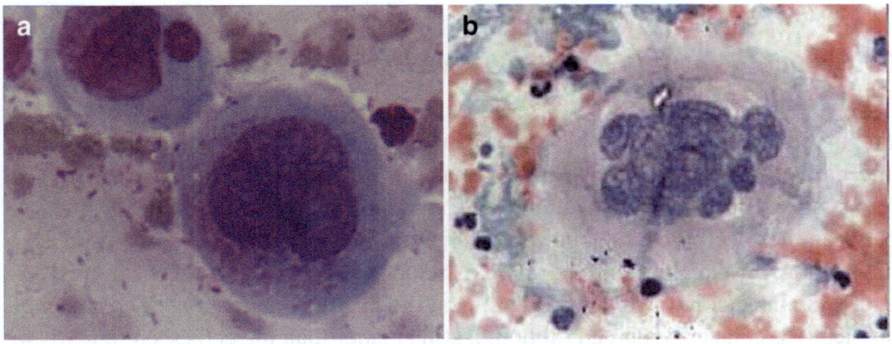

Fig. 6.7 (**a**) Radiation changes. Multinucleation and micronucleation (Giemsa, ×1,000). (**b**) Nuclear budding (H & E ×1,000). (Mehrotra R, Gupta A, Singh M, Ibrahim R. Application of cytology in diagnosing premalignant or malignant oral lesions. Mol Cancer 2006; 5: 1)

(3) Radiation and Chemotherapy Induced Oral Cytological Changes

The cytology of radiation change is similar to that described in the Pap test. There is enlargement of both the cytoplasm and the nucleus, leading to large cells termed macrocytes (Fig. 6.7a). However, the N:C ratio remains unchanged [23]. Nuclear alterations such as nuclear budding, micronucleaton and multinucleation may be seen (Fig. 6.7b) [24, 25]. Radiation also results in reactive cellular alterations, e.g. repair as discussed previously.

In a study comparing post-radiation changes in normal and malignant oral cells, it was found that various morphological abnormalities demonstrated a consistent significant increase with radiation dose [26]. Similar changes are expected to be induced by chemotherapeutic agents [27].

Atypical Changes

Atypical squamous cell alterations belong to a spectrum of cellular morphological changes which fall between normal limits or reactive on the one end, and frankly dysplastic process (indicative of a squamous intraepithelial lesion—SIL) on the other end. Reasons for the atypical diagnosis include lack of specific cytologic features or insufficient number of cells with characteristic cytologic features.

Since any meaningful classification should bear a close correlation to the biological behavior of its respective lesions and since the current guidelines for the treatment of oral dysplastic lesions advocate active treatment of high grade dysplasias [28], which are more likely to be aneuploid [29] with high risk of progression to squamous cell carcinomas [30], the term atypical is further subcategorized to illustrate the probabilities of low grade/reactive and high grade lesions.

C: Atypical Probably Reactive/Low Grade (Atypical-RL)

The atypical-RL cells resemble superficial cells, intermediate cells, reactive cells and the cells observed in low grade squamous intraepithelial lesions (LSILs), in terms of size, cytoplasmic volume and staining characteristics. The distinction between these cell types is somewhat subjective and is primarily based on nuclear morphology. It may therefore be wise to include LSIL as a subcategory in this category, the inclusion of which has no clinical/therapeutic implications. The nuclei of atypical-RL cells are enlarged (although still smaller than the cells seen in LSIL so that the N:C ratio is less than 3:1) and possess slightly irregular or smooth nuclear membranes. The nuclei are mildly hyperchromatic or hypochromatic and do not demonstrate the coarse granularity often seen in LSIL. The presence of acute inflammatory cells may favor a reactive change rather than a dysplastic process (Fig. 6.8a, b).

Low-Grade Squamous Intraepithelial Lesion

The cells of low-grade squamous intraepithelial lesion (LGSIL) are large with fairly abundant “mature” well-defined cytoplasm. As mentioned, the cytoplasmic volume and staining characteristics are similar to those of intermediate and superficial cells.

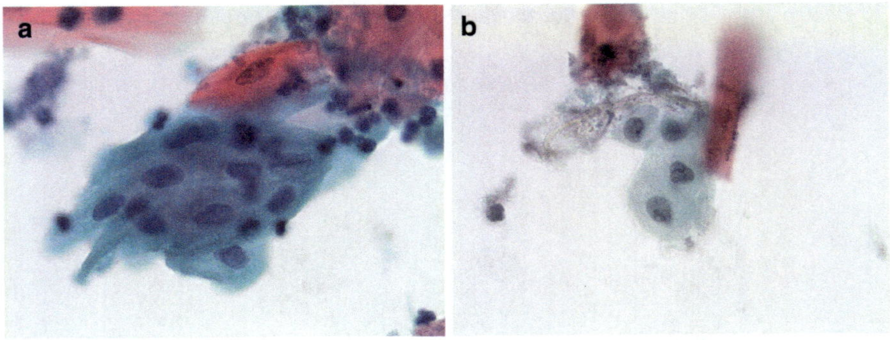

Fig. 6.8 (**a**) LBC (PapSpin). Atypical-reactive/low-grade. The cells in this image show nuclear enlargement with an attendant increase in N:C ratio, compared with the normal intermediate cell nucleus seen top right. The cells demonstrate irregularities of nuclear contours. The cytoplasm looks slightly immature (denser). Some neutrophil polymorphs are noted. The cell with the bright orangeophilic cytoplasm exhibits a degenerate nucleus. The presence of inflammatory cells favors a reactive process but a low grade squamous intraepithelial lesion cannot be completely excluded (Pap stain, ×1,000). (**b**) Atypical-reactive/low-grade. The nuclei are mildly enlarged with slight nuclear membrane irregularities; however, the nuclei are normochromatic (Pap stain, ×1,000)

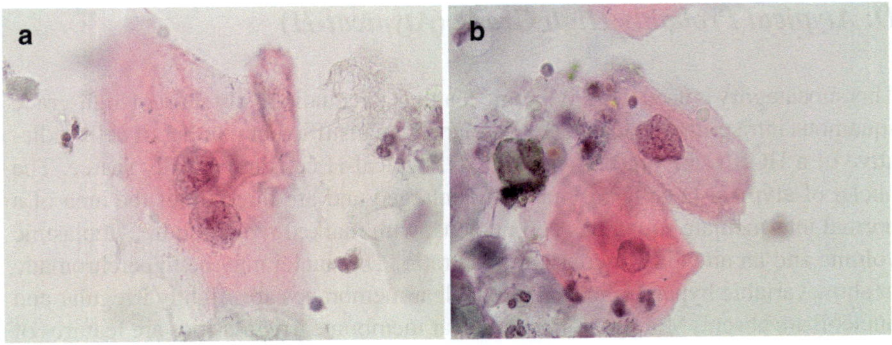

Fig. 6.9 (**a**) LBC (PapSpin). LGSIL. A large binucleated cell is seen in this image with markedly enlarged nuclei and abundant cytoplasm with a slight increase in N:C ratio. Slight irregularity of the nuclear membrane is seen. The chromatin is coarsely granular and evenly distributed. No nucleoli are identified (Pap stain, ×1,000). (**b**) A large cell is seen in the center with cytomorphological features of LSIL (×1,000)

These cells often standout at screening magnification. Large hyperchromatic nuclei are seen, three times the size of the intermediate cell nuclei, which results in a slightly increased N:C ratio. Slight irregularities of the nuclear membranes are visible. The chromatin is coarsely granular and uniformly spread. Nucleoli are not a feature of LGSIL (Fig. 6.9a, b).

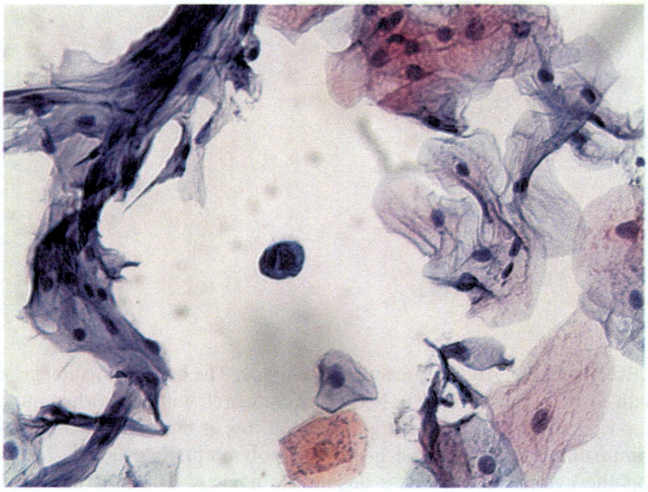

Fig. 6.10 LBC (SurePath). Atypical/high-grade. A single cell is seen in the center with enlarged and intensely hyperchromatic nucleus. The scanty cytoplasm results in a high N:C ratio. The nuclear membrane outline is strikingly irregular. The cytomorphology is that of a HGSIL, however, because this is the only cell observed, the diagnosis was limited to Atypical/high-grade (Pap stain, ×400)

D: Atypical Probably High Grade (Atypical-H)

This subcategory is used if the cytologic features fall qualitatively short of high-grade squamous intraepithelial lesion (HGSIL), or if an insufficient number of cells indicative of a HGSIL are present (Fig. 6.10). Atypical-H cells are usually scarce. The nuclei of atypical-H cells are markedly enlarged and are three times the area of a normal intermediate squamous cell nucleus, with marked reduction in cytoplasmic volume and an attendant increase in N:C ratio. The nuclei may be hyperchromatic or show variable hyperchromasia; the nuclear membranes are slightly irregular and nucleoli are absent. More prominent nuclear membrane irregularities are features of a HGSIL.

E: High-Grade Squamous Intraepithelial Lesion

The cells of high-grade squamous intraepithelial lesion (HGSIL) may be arranged as single cells, streaming sheets or syncytial clusters. A syncytium is a three dimensional group of closely packed and haphazardly arranged hyperchromatic nuclei with molding. No cell borders can be perceived. Mitotic figures and apoptotic bodies can be seen in large syncytial clusters.

The cells of HGSIL possess markedly enlarged and hyperchromatic nuclei (which may be the same size or less than that of a LSIL) with scanty dense cytoplasm and

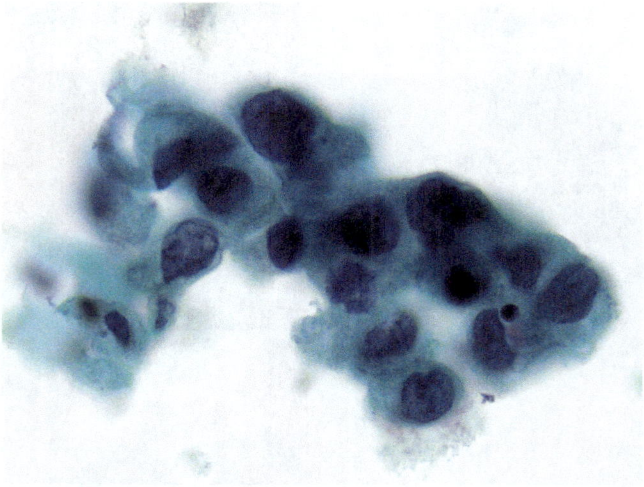

Fig. 6.11 LBC (PapSpin). HGSIL—In this high grade lesion, the cells show high N:C ratios and nuclear hyperchromasia with coarsely granular chromatin. The nuclear membranes are irregular, and the cytoplasm has a hard (dense) appearance (Pap stain, ×1,000)

thus a very high N:C ratio. Irregularities of nuclear contour are striking, especially in liquid-based preparations. The chromatin pattern is finely or coarsely granular but is uniformly distributed. Nucleoli are not seen (Fig. 6.11).

F: Invasive Squamous Cell Carcinoma

In invasive squamous cell carcinoma (SCC) the cells are found as syncytial groups. Pronounced nuclear alterations are features of invasive SCC and include marked variation in nuclear shape and size, irregularities of nuclear membrane, prominent irregular nucleoli, variably sized and irregularly distributed chromatin clumps separated by areas of clearing (Fig. 6.12a). There is often shedding of isolated single cells with malignant nuclear features.

In keratinizing squamous cell carcinomas, there is usually evidence of atypical keratin pearls. (Fig. 6.12b) Occasionally some malignant cells may display a cannibalistic behavior ("Cell in Cell"—Fig. 6.12c) and abnormally configured keratotic cells with bizarre shapes (spindling, tadpole shapes or long cytoplasmic projections—(Figs. 6.12d and 6.13a, b). The abnormal keratotic cells are evidence of abnormal maturation and possess dense orange/blue or pink cytoplasm and intensely hyperchromatic nuclei. Although they are often associated with an invasive SCC, they may be encountered in non-invasive lesions, and the correct

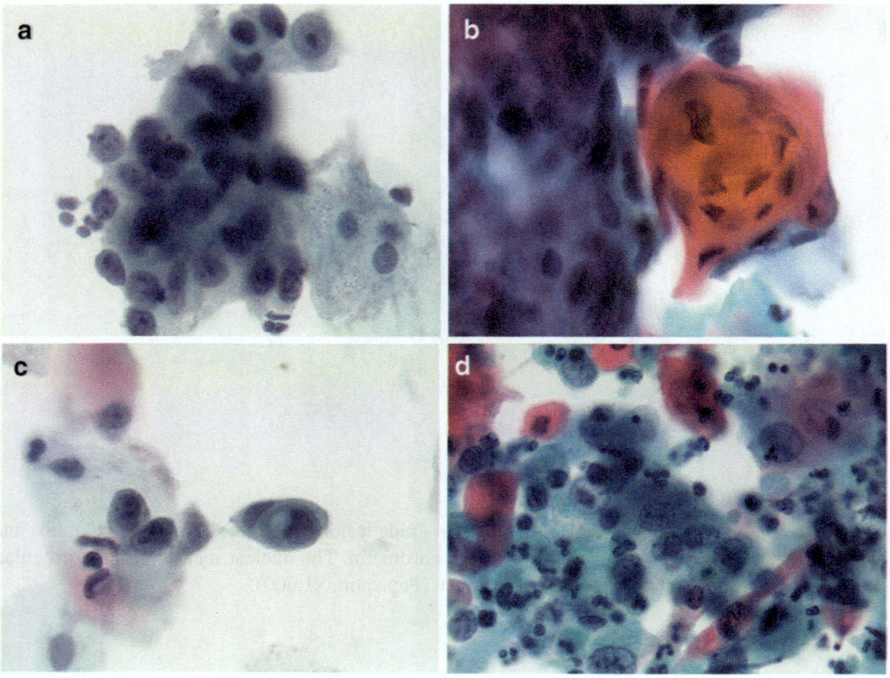

Fig. 6.12 (**a**) LBC (PapSpin). Invasive squamous cell carcinoma-haphazard arrangement of variably sized cells in syncytial arrangement typical of carcinoma. This contrasts with the streaming arrangement seen in repair. The nuclei demonstrate chromatin clearing, prominent irregular nucleoli and irregular nuclear outlines (Pap stain, ×1,000). (**b**) Invasive squamous cell carcinoma—an atypical keratin pearl, pathognomonic of keratinizing squamous cell carcinoma (Pap stain, ×1,000). (**c**) Invasive squamous cell carcinoma—"cell in cell" (cannibalism) (Pap stain, ×1,000). (**d**) Invasive squamous cell carcinoma—In addition to the carcinoma cells this image shows an abnormally configured keratotic cell with long cytoplasmic projections, bright pink cytoplasm, and intensely hyperchromatic irregular nucleus (*bottom right*). A parakeratotic cell and an abnormal cytoplasmic fragment are seen on the left (Pap stain, ×1,000)

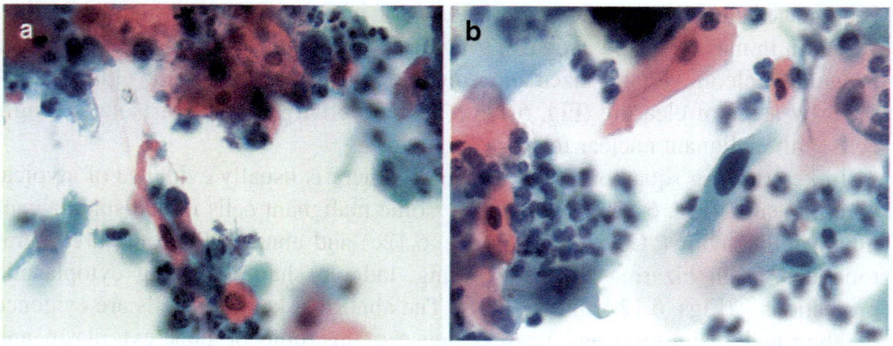

Fig. 6.13 (**a**, **b**) LBC (PapSpin). Abnormally configured spindled keratotic cells and small parakeratotic cells (Pap stain, ×1,000)

interpretation of carcinoma is based on the presence of nuclear abnormalities described, identified by careful study of numerous cells and cell groups.

The background may show necrosis, which may occasionally collect at the periphery of the cell groups (clinging necrosis) and a scattering of (abnormal) cytoplasmic fragments. The syncytial arrangement of carcinoma cells, together with their prominent nucleoli and nuclear pallor (clearing) may simulate repair, however, the finding of flat, streaming cohesive sheets of cells in repair contrasts the haphazard arrangement of cells in invasive SCC. In addition, no single cells with malignant nuclear features are identified in repair and the chromatin remains pale, uniform and finely granular.

Verrucous Carcinoma

The diagnosis of verrucous carcinoma can only be made on histologic sections that are deep enough to demonstrate the downward pushing epithelium in relation to the underlying submucosa. Generally there is no evidence of cellular atypia in the absence of malignant transformation/invasion and hence the cytological features of verrucous carcinoma are non-specific; they usually demonstrate abundant parakeratosis and unremarkable epithelial cells.

Future Perspectives

While still at its infancy, this grading system provides a standardized and uniform method of reporting for the practising oral pathologist. To further validate the newly proposed classification scheme and discover the best cut-off value for distinguishing reactive/low grade lesions from high grade/squamous cell carcinoma, the authors propose a simple and easy scoring method based on nine cytologic characteristics [19] which may well increase the specificity of the oral cytology test in a manner similar to that of the Pap test (Table 6.2). It was found that a cytologic score of <3 indicated a reactive/low grade lesion and a cytologic score of 3 or more indicated a high grade lesion or invasive squamous cell carcinoma, with high sensitivity (95%) and specificity (96%) (Fig. 6.14).

While the newly proposed oral cytologic scoring system shows promise to be simple, reliable and reproducible, future large scale studies including an acceptable large number of clinical Class I lesions (clinically worrisome that would typically raise suspicion for premalignancy or invasive cancer) and Class II lesions (primarily not strongly suspicious for a high-grade dysplasia or an invasive carcinoma and would otherwise not trigger an invasive diagnostic procedure) will have to confirm its applicability and usefulness and determine the optimal score for each cytologic diagnostic category. This is ideally achieved through prospective multicenter

Table 6.2 Oral/oropharyngeal cytologic scoring system

Scoring system	
Irregular nuclear membrane	Yes (1)/No (0)
Irregular chromatin distribution/hyperchromasia	Yes (1)/No (0)
Prominent nucleoli	Yes (1)/No (0)
Abnormal cell shapes[a]	Yes (1)/No (0)
Parakeratotic cells[b]	Yes (1)/No (0)
Necrosis	Yes (1)/No (0)
Syncytial groups (>10 cells)[c]	Yes (1)/No (0)
Irregular nucleoli	Yes (1)/No (0)
Abnormal cytoplasmic fragments	Yes (1)/No (0)

[a]Abnormal cell shapes: Abnormally configured keratotic cells with spindling, tadpole shapes or long cytoplasmic projections

[b]Parakeratotic Cells: Cells with dense orangeophilic cytoplasm and small hyperchromatic degenerate nuclei. The nuclear-to-cytoplasmic ratio is low

[c]Syncytial groups: Pleomorphic cells seen in three-dimensional clusters

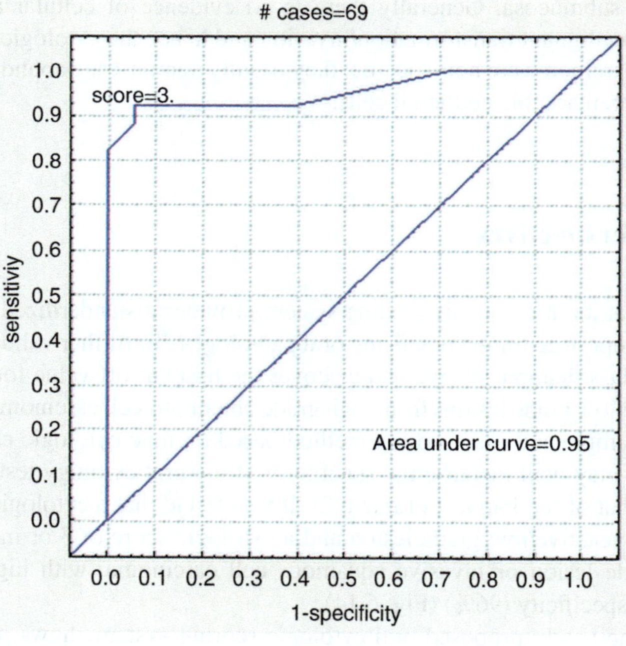

Fig. 6.14 A score of 3 was found to be the optimal cut-off value to discriminate between reactive/ low-grade and high-grade/invasive SCC

collaborative studies in oral cancer screening with possible application of molecular diagnostics and immunocytochemistry for detection of predictive cellular antigens (e.g. D2-40/Podoplanin—Fig. 6.15).

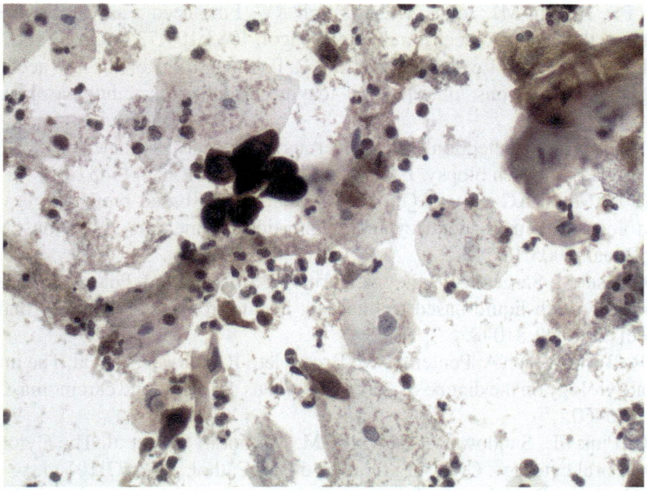

Fig. 6.15 D2-40 (Podoplanin) immunocytochemistry. This image shows strong staining of tumor cells, weak to moderate staining of dysplastic cells and lack of staining of reactive and normal intermediate, and superficial cells (×400)

Acknowledgements Prof CA Wright, Dr PT Schubert and Mrs G Neethling, Cytology unit, Division of Anatomical Pathology, University of Stellenbosch and NHLS Tygerberg, Cape Town, South Africa.

References

1. Papanicolaou GN, Traut HF. The diagnostic value of vaginal smears in carcinoma of the uterus. Am J Obstet Gynecol. 1941;42:193–206.
2. National Cancer Institute Workshop. The 1988 Bethesda System for reporting cervical/vaginal cytologic diagnoses. JAMA. 1989;262:931–4.
3. Reagan JW, Seidemann IL, Saracusa Y. The cellular morphology of carcinoma in situ and dysplasia or atypical hyperplasia of the uterine cervix. Cancer. 1953;6:224–35.
4. Koss LG. Diagnostic cytology and its histopathologic bases. 4th ed. Philadelphia: J.B. Lipincott Co; 1992.
5. Richart RM. Natural history of cervical intraepithelial neoplasia. Clin Obstet Gynecol. 1967;10:748–84.
6. The Bethesda System for reporting cervical/vaginal cytologic diagnoses: report of the 1991 Bethesda Workshop. JAMA. 1992; 267: 1892.
7. Solomon D, Davey DD, Kurman R, et al. The 2001 Bethesda System: terminology for reporting results of cervical cytology. JAMA. 2002;287:2114–9.
8. Nichols ML, Quinn FB, Schnadig VJ, Zaharopoulos P, Hokanson JA, Des Jardins L, et al. Interobserver variability in the interpretation of brush cytologic studies from head and neck lesions. Arch Otolaryngol Head Neck Surg. 1991;117:1350–5.
9. Kaugars GE, Silverman S, Ray AK, Page DG, Abbey LM, Burns JC, et al. The use of exfoliative cytology for the early diagnosis of oral cancers: is there a role for it in education and private practice? J Cancer Educ. 1998;13:85–9.

10. Feldman PS, Kaplan MJ, Johns ME, Cantrell RW. Fine-needle aspiration in squamous cell carcinoma of the head and neck. Arch Otolaryngol. 1983;109:735–42.
11. Scher RL, Oostingh PE, Levine PA, Cantrell R, Feldman PS. Role of fine needle aspiration in the diagnosis of lesions of the oral cavity, oropharynx, and nasopharynx. Cancer. 1988;62:2602–6.
12. Sciubba JJ. Improving detection of precancerous and cancerous oral lesions: computer-assisted analysis of the oral brush biopsy. J Am Dent Assoc. 1999;130:1445–57.
13. Hayama FH, Motta AC, Silva AG, Migliari DA. Liquid-based preparations versus conventional cytology: specimen adequacy and diagnostic agreement in oral lesions. Med Oral Patol Oral Cir Bucal. 2005;10:115–22.
14. Kujan O, Desai M, Sargent A, Bailey A, Turner A, Sloan P, et al. Potential applications of oral brush cytology with liquid-based technology: results from a cohort of normal oral mucosa. Oral Oncol. 2006;42:810–8.
15. Navone R, Burlo P, Pich A, Pentenero M, Broccoletti R, Marsico A, et al. The impact of liquid-based oral cytology on the diagnosis of oral squamous dysplasia and carcinoma. Cytopathology. 2007;18:356–60.
16. Jones AC, Pink FE, Sandow PL, Stewart CM, Migliorati CA, et al. The Cytobrush Plus cell collector in oral cytology. Oral Surg Oral Med Oral Pathol. 1994;77:101–4.
17. Driemel O, Dashe R, Hakim G, Tsioutsias T, Pistner H, Reichert TE, Kosmehl H. Laminin-5 immunocytochemistry: a new tool for identifying dysplastic cells in oral brush biopsies. Cytopathology. 2007;18:348–55.
18. Hutchinson ML, Isenstein LM, Goodman A, Hurley AA, Douglass KL, Mui KK, et al. Homogeneous sampling accounts for the increased diagnostic accuracy using the Thin Prep processor. Am J Clin Pathol. 1994;101:215–9.
19. Afrogheh A, Wright CA, Sellars SL, Pelsar A, Wetter J, Schubert PT, Hille J. An evaluation of the Shandon PapSpin liquid based oral test utilizing a novel cytologic scoring system. Oral Surg Oral Med Oral Pathol. 2012;113:799–807.
20. Solomon D, Nayar R, editors. The Bethesda system for reporting cervical cytology. 2nd ed. New York: Springer; 2004.
21. Christian DC. Computer-assisted of oral brush biopsies at and oral cancer screening program. J Am Dent Assoc. 2002;133:357–62.
22. Drinnan AJ. Screening for oral cancer and precancer – a valuable new technique. Gen Dent. 2000;48:656–60.
23. Ogden GR, Cowpe JG, Green MW. Effect of radiotherapy on oral mucosa assessed by quantitative exfoliative cytology. J Clin Pathol. 1989;42:940–3.
24. Bhattathiri NV, Bharathykkutty C, Prathapan R, et al. Prediction of radiosensitivity of oral cancers by serial cytological assay of nuclear changes. Radiother Oncol. 1998;49:61–5.
25. Bhattathiri N, Bindu L, Remani P, et al. Radiation induced acute immediate nuclear abnormalities in oral cancer cells: serial cytologic evaluation. Acta Cytol. 1998;42:1084–90.
26. Mehrotra R, Madhu R, Singh M. Serial scrape smear cytology of radiation response in normal and malignant cells of oral cavity. Indian J Pathol Microbiol. 2004;47:497–502.
27. Koss LG. Cytologic diagnosis of oral, esophageal, and peripheral lung cancer. J Cell Biochem. 1993;17F(Suppl):66–81.
28. Van der Waal I. Potentially malignant disorders of the oral and oropharyngeal mucosa; terminology, classification and present concepts of management. Oral Oncol. 2009;45:317–23.
29. Hirshberg A, Yarom N, Amariglio N, et al. Detection of non-diploid cells in premalignant and malignant oral lesions using combined morphological and FISH analysis-a new method for early detection of suspicious oral lesions. Cancer Lett. 2007;253:282–90.
30. Torres-Rendon A, Stewart R, Craig CT, Wells M, Speight PM. DNA ploidy analysis by image cytometry helps to identify oral epithelial dysplasias with high risk of malignant progression. Oral Oncol. 2009;45:468–73.

Chapter 7
Liquid-Based Oral Cytology and Microhistology

Roberto Navone, Monica Pentenero, and Sergio Gandolfo

Oral squamous cell carcinoma (OSCC) is a frequently encountered malignant lesion and still occupies the sixth or seventh place in cancer-related mortality worldwide. Even if approximately 75% of the cases occur in the developing world, with a high mortality rate [1], the more developed countries are still greatly affected. Indeed, it has been estimated that over 40% of lesions of the oropharyngeal cavity out of the 643,000 newly diagnosed cases of head and neck malignancies annually are carcinomas. The Italian tumor registry [2] reports 2,978 deaths, with a 38% global and 44% relative 5 year-survival rate. Although this type of cancer is closely related to lifestyle, such as tobacco and alcohol consumption, there are also other major risk factors, which may also be genetic and/or viral [3, 4]. Unfortunately, the last 30 years have not witnessed any significant improvement in survival rate and less than 50% of patients with oropharyngeal cancer achieve 5-year survival. This is most likely due to the fact that this type of tumor is, more often than not, diagnosed at an advanced stage, resulting in a high relapse rate as well as the increased incidence of second tumors in patients with head and neck OSCC. Moreover, a significant increase in OSCC [5] has recently been reported by numerous European countries, such as the U.K., France and Eastern Europe. A study carried out in India [6] has demonstrated that screening programs, based on periodic objective oral cavity

R. Navone (✉)
Department of Biomedical Sciences and Human Oncology, Pathology Section, University of Turin, via Santena 7, 10126 Torino, Italy

Anatomia Patologica, University of Turin, via Santena 7, 10126 Torino, Italy
e-mail: Roberto.navone@unito.it

M. Pentenero • S. Gandolfo
Department of Clinical and Biological Sciences, Oral Medicine and Oral Oncology Section, University of Turin, Regione Gonzole 10, 10043 Orbassano (Torino), Italy

R. Mehrotra (ed.), *Oral Cytology: A Concise Guide*, DOI 10.1007/978-1-4614-5221-8_7,

visual examination, are able to reduce the OSCC mortality rate in high risk individuals. However, to date, there is insufficient validated data on programs based not only on oral cavity examination but also on other parameters (like exfoliative cytology). In 2010, the American Dental Association Council on Scientific Affairs Expert Panel on Screening for Oral Squamous Cell Carcinomas stated: "Additional research regarding oral cancer screening and the use of adjuncts is needed" [7]. In fact, at the time of writing, although numerous reviews have dealt with the role of oral cytology and other techniques for the diagnosis and/or the screening of OSCC and/or OPML [8–12], but conclusive data is still lacking.

Indeed, as many OSCC are either preceded or accompanied by precursor lesions, such as OPML, especially leukoplakia, or erythroplakia, the easy access to oral mucosa for clinical examination offers an outstanding advantage for early diagnosis and prevention. As the lesions of oral precancer and early cancer are usually asymptomatic, they may be "a chance finding", or occasionally observed during routine dental visits, or treatment. Nevertheless, the high prevalence of oral abnormalities observed during a routine dental visit [13] makes it impractical for the dental practitioner to refer every oral lesion to specialized centers for scalpel biopsy and histological evaluation. Indeed, the referral of all the detected lesions to specialized centers is not only time consuming but also implies an increase in both patient anxiety and costs, making it basically an unfair use of national health service resources. This, however, could well lead to an increase in the diagnostic delay, which is a key issue in oral oncology.

Furthermore, a contributing factor to the poor prognosis of oral neoplasia may well be the very fact that the definitive diagnosis of the OSCC and its precursors (dysplasia) is still mainly based on scalpel biopsy. In fact, although this invasive technique poses sampling limits, as it can be carried out only in restricted areas and on a limited number of sites, it remains the most commonly used technique worldwide. These limits make for an insufficient sampling of multiple lesions, even if it is well known that even a single lesion amongst many, or, indeed even only *a small part* of a single lesion, may show microscopic evidence of malignancy, or dysplasia, which may be overlooked by the traditional scalpel biopsy.

Moreover, not all oral lesions observed are routinely biopsied, as surgery is generally reserved for only the so-called class I lesions—i.e. those with high clinical suspicion. These lesions are typically in advanced stages; however, false negative rates can be as high as 23% even in the strongly suspicious lesions [14]. There is an evident need for a reliable and repeatable first level test to identify *all* the lesions that, due to their morphologic and/or molecular characteristics, must be further investigated with a second level test, i.e. with a scalpel (surgical) biopsy. The availability of such a test is particularly important for the oral lesions which look apparently innocent on clinical examination (class II) that would not, as aforementioned, be routinely biopsied. This is already the case in screening of carcinoma of the uterine cervix, where the Papanicolaou (Pap) test and colposcopy with biopsy meet these requirements. Indeed, the Pap test is a well-known and accepted efficacious first level examination that has been demonstrated to reduce both the incidence and mortality rate of cervical carcinoma, as it identifies intraepithelial pre-neoplastic (dysplastic) lesions so that they may be treated, *before* they evolve into invasive (malignant) forms. However, despite diagnostic oral cytology having been well known now for many years and the fact that it is a simple, non-invasive, painless, inexpensive technique which may be applied even to extensive and multiple lesions, to date, it has not yet been as widely adopted as a first level test, as has cervico-vaginal cytology. Paradoxically, it seems that a pelvic examination, or Pap smear, is *more socially acceptable* [15] than are examinations of the oral cavity, a point of view shared by both patients and physicians alike. This means that a significant number of early oral lesions are missed by patients and/or healthcare professionals [15]. Consequently, most OSCC remain undetected until a late stage, making the overall percentage of diagnosis of localized oral cancers similar to that of cancer of the colon (36%), which is somewhat surprising as an evaluation of the colon mucosa requires quite a laborious and somewhat forbidding endoscopic examination [15].

The frequent incidental finding (by conventional oral examination) of oral mucosal lesions makes it important that examination should be combined with an effective first level diagnostic test so as to select lesions that require further evaluation in specialized centers e.g. hospitals or universities, as does the Pap test for cervical cancer. To this aim, a more extensive use of oral diagnostic cytology had been proposed, as cytology is a practical, quick, uncomplicated, painless, cost-efficient, non-invasive, repeatable technique, which can also be used for multiple lesions. Furthermore, some recent reports indicate that both the efficacy and efficiency of oral cytology may be enhanced by the use of new ancillary techniques thus ensuring an increase in sensitivity and specificity. These new approaches include: liquid-based cytology, brush biopsy cytology and computer-assisted cytology (Oral CDx), immunocytochemistry, flow and image cytometry, molecular biology and, last but not least, the so-called microhistology. The next section will discuss the various options in more detail, along with the authors' personal experience on the field.

Conventional Oral Cytology

The use of exfoliative oral diagnostic cytology was quite common in the 1960s and 1970s. Indeed, it was in this period that Allegra et al. [16] reported on a large study population of 6,448 oral cytology specimens, diagnosing 74 carcinomas with only two false negatives. There was, however, a bias in these data as histology was performed exclusively in positive and/or suspicious cytology cases and not in the presence of a negative result. Unfortunately, since then oral conventional cytology has lost a lot of ground, even if it is still used in some centers [17, 18] and has been the basis of few studies on morphometric differences between normal and neoplastic cells [19]. The responsibility for this drop in popularity may be attributed to a number of factors, such as diagnostic/interpretative difficulties and/or the sampling technique itself, which are not to be underestimated. The fact that many oral lesions have resistant, keratotic surfaces also makes a negative contribution—as this means that samples are often inadequate due to their being too superficial and/or bloody.

Liquid-Based Cytology

A relatively recent method has been introduced, which, to date, has mainly been used for the Pap test, i.e. liquid-based cytology. This technique has given promising results, both in terms of sample quality, as there are no cellular artifacts and in terms of quantity, that is to say it is possible to analyze practically *all* the cells collected and there are fewer inadequate cases. Navone et al. [20] studied 473 patients with a suspicion of OSCC, or OPML referred to the Oral Medicine Section of the University of Turin for a scalpel biopsy. After sampling for cytology, all patients, whether cytologically positive or negative, underwent a surgical biopsy and the specimens were examined histologically. Conventional cytology was used to process 89/473 samples and 384 were processed using liquid-based cytology (Thin Prep). Whereas, conventional oral cytology gave 12.4% of inadequate cases, liquid-based cytology gave 8.8%; the sensitivity, specificity, predictive positive value and predictive negative values were 85.7%, 95.9%, 95.4% and 87.0%, respectively, for conventional samples, versus 95.1%, 99.0%, 96.3% and 98.7% for liquid-based cytology. This study demonstrated that conventional oral cytology has a better sensitivity and positive predictive value than the conventional cervical smear test (Pap test), whilst its specificity is similar. Both the sensitivity and specificity were better in oral liquid-based than in conventional cytology and there were fewer inadequate samples.

These results were supported by other authors reporting similar data: e.g. Delavarian et al. [21] who studied 25 patients and obtained values of 88.8%, 100.0%, 100.0% and 80.0%. One report [22] dealing with healthy volunteers was done to demonstrate the potential applications of liquid-based oral cytology in different fields. Other authors [23] published smaller cohorts, without data on sensitivity or specificity. However, these papers differ in the strategy applied by Navone et al. [20], in as much as no histological examinations of cases with a negative cytological diagnosis were carried out.

To the best of our knowledge, the only other research involving the use of the oral brush and scalpel biopsies performed simultaneously on patients with minimally suspicious oral lesions (Class II lesions) is that by Mehrotra et al. [24]. A total of 85 patients were enrolled and demonstrated a 100% specificity for the "positive" cases and 90.4% for "atypical" case with a 96.3% sensitivity in both groups.

There are various factors that make an early diagnosis of oral carcinoma far from easy: however, the application of innovative technologies as the use of liquid-based instead of conventional cytology may help to resolve some of these problems. However, diagnostic oral exfoliative cytology is labor intensive, requires a high degree of expertise for the identification and evaluation of cells with "atypical morphology" and has been reported to be insufficiently sensitive, at least for pre-invasive OPML, by some authors [11]. Cells exfoliated from oral mucosa, such as the samples used for liquid-based cytology, could be used for the analysis of the molecular alterations that could be more objective and aim at the identification of specific gene-related anomalies [9]. However, the road which may establish exactly how useful these techniques are, either alone or in association with oral cytology, for early detection of OSCC and the risk of their evolving into OPML, is still long and uncertain. The most reasonable approach might well be to make a critical analysis of more first-level tests, as liquid-based cytology, non-invasive microbiopsies (described in detail further on), DNA analysis, etc., to assess their ability to identify dysplastic/neoplastic cells or DNA alterations which could be an indication for histological confirmation by scalpel biopsy.

DNA Analysis with Flow and Image Cytometry

As it has been reported that DNA cellular content i.e. ploidy, is a reliable marker in oral oncology for both malignant and premalignant lesions, DNA ploidy has been studied both by flow and image cytometry. Samples obtained using the liquid-based cytology method seems to be particularly suitable for this aim. Flow cytometry was used on oral samples by Marsico et al. [25] to examine 211 OPML diagnosed by scalpel biopsy. Flow cytometry demonstrated aneuploidy i.e. an abnormal number of chromosomes, in 24/40 (60.0%) OSCC, in 16/70 (22.8%) of the OPML without dysplasia and in 17/30 (56.7%) of the OPML with dysplasia. Pentenero et al. [26] demonstrated that the DNA aneuploidy and dysplasia observed in 60 OPML were strictly associated with cigarette smoking and site of the lesion and Donadini et al. [27], studying 109 OPML, observed the prevalence of single near-diploid sublines in non-dysplastic OPML, whereas multiple highly aneuploid sublines were widespread in dysplastic OPML and OSCC. Similar results were obtained in oral verrucous carcinomas [28].

The near-diploid aneuploidy in OPML seemed to be early events of oral carcinogenesis, in agreement with the concept of "field cancerization" [29, 30]. Torres-Rendon et al. [31] observed aneuploidy in 14/42 (33.3%) of OPML that progressed to OSCC, but in only 5/44 (11.3%) of OPML that did not progress. The sensitivity and specificity of image cytometry in detecting cases with high risk of malignant progression was 0.33 and 0.88 respectively [31].

Microhistology: "The Curette Technique"

With the aim of increasing the quantity of cells available for cytological examination and the other complementary techniques, Navone et al. [32–35] set up, and applied, a new sampling technique that was no longer based on the use of a "Cytobrush", but rather on "scraping" the oral mucosa with a dermatological curette. Right from the very first sampling, it was evident that not only did this technique provide more abundant material for cytology and ploidy [20, 25–28], but that the samples were richer *in "accidentally acquired" small fragments*, that we decided to further investigate as *micro-biopsies (micro-histology)*.

As a rule, no local anesthesia is used and topical sprays or emulsions/creams should be avoided as lubrication of the lesion surface reduces scraping efficacy when collecting tissue fragments. Scraping is to be carried out on the whole of the surface of the oral lesion, taking care to provoke a slight bleeding to ensure sampling of the basal layers of the epithelium. The curette is held tangential to the lesion surface to avoid cutting rather than scraping. The scraping is to be continued until such times as an adequate amount of tissue fragments have been obtained (usually from 20 to 40 times, depending on the site and clinical aspect of the lesion). The lesion is to be kept free from saliva/blood with gauze to maximize scraping efficacy. The material obtained is placed into a fixing liquid in a vial, which can be gently shaken to visually ensure adequacy. The technique is minimally invasive and, differently from traditional scalpel biopsy, is able to cover the whole surface of the lesion.

These micro-biopsies are then embedded in paraffin, cut with a microtome, stained with hematoxylin-eosin and subjected to routine histological examination. No dedicated technical devices, other than those used routinely in a pathology lab, are necessary. A sample may be considered adequate when it contains at least 100 non-superficial cells on a representative strip of epithelium, whilst, when only horny material (anucleated cells) is present, it is defined as inadequate [32].

From a pathological point of view, the reduced dimensions of the micro-biopsy samples and their lack of orientation may imply some disadvantages e.g. it may be difficult to recognize the invasiveness of high grade lesions. Nonetheless, this may be considered of minor importance in a first level diagnostic test where the aim is to detect any sign of dysplastic/malignant alteration - whatever the grade. In this way, all oral lesions, including those with the lowest suspicion index, can be examined by cytology and microhistology, as well as by conventional (scalpel biopsy) histology, for an early identification of cancerous and/or precancerous oral lesions. Indeed, there was a very low inadequacy sample rate with the microhistology technique (3.66%). This implies that microhistology is neither a difficult nor a demanding procedure to master—an element of utmost importance when considering the fact that a first level technique is usually in the hands of dental practitioners, who, though experts in their own field, have no specialist training in oncology. In fact, no particular competence is required to perform the micro-biopsy, nor is it necessary to make a comprehensive analysis of the clinical aspect of the lesion. Moreover, as this technique offers the possibility of sampling large areas, there is no need to choose a very specific site. Our previous research has demonstrated that microhistology is highly reliable in the detection of oncological alterations as a first-level test in suspicious lesions assessed by oral medicine practitioners [34]. At present, further research on the feasibility of the general dentist carrying out microbiopsies is ongoing. As aforementioned, no dedicated laboratory equipment is required, therefore, if the results of our on-going study confirm the "user-friendly" aspect of this technique, microhistology might well represent a reliable aid for first level diagnosis also in developing countries. It goes without saying that this technique offers a valuable aid for specialists when faced with the follow-up of PML patients who object to continuous invasive histological evaluations. On the basis of the fact that there were extremely few false negatives i.e. 3/138 versus 7/138 with liquid-based cytology and 10/138 with the scalpel biopsy, later on in our study the scalpel biopsy was reserved to only positive and/or dubious cases, whilst negative cases were subjected to a strict follow-up (every 6 months).

Microhistology seems to be of particular relevance when immunohistochemistry is called for, with the aim of evaluating the risk of malignant transformation or the proliferative activity of an oral lesion. Mutation of the tumor suppressor gene p53, a marker of genomic instability associated with the cell cycle, is one of the most frequent genomic changes in human cancers. In OSCC and OPML, suprabasal p53 immunoexpression is strongly associated with high grade dysplasia and risk of malignant transformation and can also be detected in malignant cells obtained by exfoliative cytology [36, 37]. The nuclear expression of Ki67, a cell proliferation marker, may provide useful information for the evaluation of the grading of oral epithelial dysplasia and the risk of evolution into OSCC [37, 38]. The overexpression of the p16 protein, a negative regulator of the cell cycle, in OPML, may also be significant when investigating the evolution of precancerous diseases in the oral cavity [38, 39]. Even if immunocytochemistry is used on cytology samples i.e. on exfoliated oral cells, it is doubtful that the results obtained would be comparable to those obtained by histological samples. This would apply, in particular, if the investigation were to involve p53 or Ki67, where the position of the positive cells i.e. in proximity to the basal membrane, or in a suprabasal site, is of great importance. That is why these techniques can be particularly useful if associated to the microhistology.

Data on Personal Experience

The authors carried out a cytological study on oral lesions as follows:

1. From 1998 to 2005, on 411 individuals using scalpel biopsy in all cases (both positive and negative) in combination with liquid-based cytology;
2. From 2005 to 2008, on164 individuals using scalpel biopsy in all cases (both positive and negative) in combination with liquid-based cytology and microhistology;
3. From 2008 to 2011, on 252 individuals using liquid-based cytology in combination with microhistology in all cases, whilst scalpel biopsy was reserved to positive cases.

Although the data that were collected from this personal experience showed that liquid-based cytology gave good results as to sensibility and specificity, microhistology gave better results, especially as to sensitivity.

As described above:

1. Sensitivity, specificity, positive predictive value (PPV) and inadequate percentage of oral traditional cytology were 86.5%, 94.3%, 95.7% and 12.4% respectively;

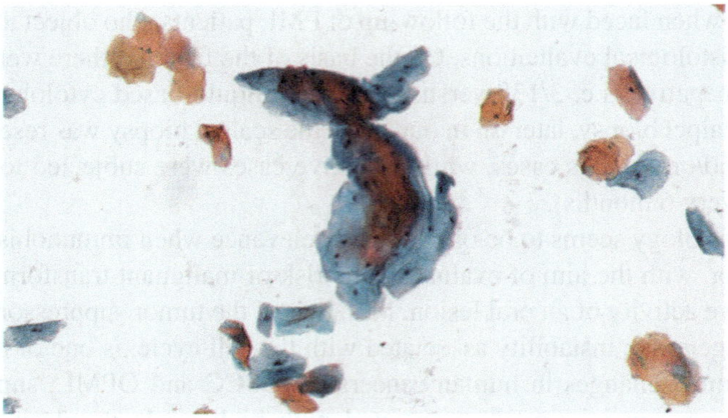

Fig. 7.1 Normal oral squamous cells and anucleated (keratotic) cells as observed in liquid-based cytology (Papanicolaou stain- mag. ×200)

2. Sensitivity, specificity, positive predictive value (PPV) and inadequate percentage of oral liquid-based cytology were 94.7%, 98.9%, 95.9% and 8.2% respectively;
3. Sensitivity, specificity, positive predictive value (PPV) and inadequate percentage of microhistology were 97.7%, 99.1%, 98.7% and 3.7% respectively;
4. Sensitivity of scalpel biopsy was only 85.9% in the paper published by Navone et al. [33].

Therefore, microhistology gave better results than liquid-based cytology or even scalpel biopsy [34, 35]. Figures 7.1, 7.2, 7.3, 7.4, 7.5, 7.6, 7.7, 7.8, 7.9, 7.10, 7.11, 7.12, 7.13, 7.14, 7.15, 7.16, 7.17, 7.18, 7.19, and 7.20 show the main characteristics of the normal/dysplastic/neoplastic oral squamous cells in liquid-based cytology and microhistology. Microhistology also allowed for immunohistochemistry investigations to be carried out on the same sample, as shown in Figs. 7.21, 7.22, 7.23, and 7.24.

Conventional, and especially liquid-based exfoliative cytology, is able to provide satisfactory diagnostic information. The sensitivity of oral cytology is higher than that of the cervico-vaginal (Pap test), whilst its specificity is the same. Although the number of inadequate cases is still, at time of writing, too high, we are of the opinion that it can be reduced. "Ancillary" techniques, such as flow and/or image cytometry for DNA, allow for the detection of aneuploid OPML in the absence of dysplasia by conventional histology, i.e. the identification of lesions that are at risk of evolution, such as that which the search for specific markers with immunocytochemistry and molecular analysis is able to provide. Sampling with the "curette technique", which covers ample surface areas and/or multiple lesions and provides "microbiopsies", make for a reduction in the number of patients that are obliged to return for further investigation, as well as in the number of diagnostic (scalpel) biopsies that have to be carried out, leading to a positive cost/benefit ratio for the hospital structure and less discomfort/anxiety for the patient. Moreover, this relatively simple and "patient/user friendly" technique make it a good candidate for application not only for ENT specialists, but also in the field of general dentistry, as

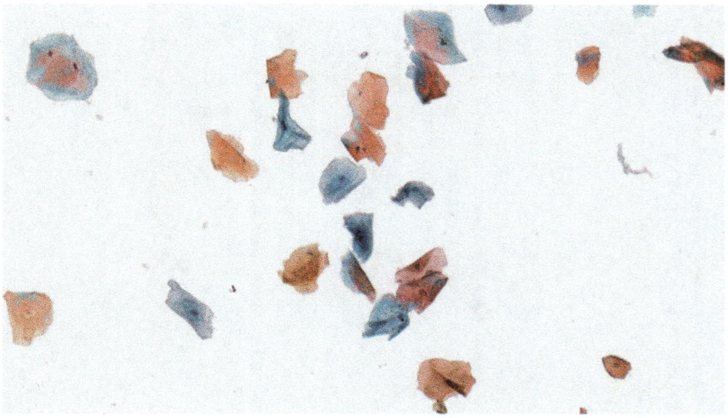

Fig. 7.2 Normal oral squamous cells and anucleated (keratotic) cells as observed in liquid-based cytology (Papanicolaou stain- mag. ×200)

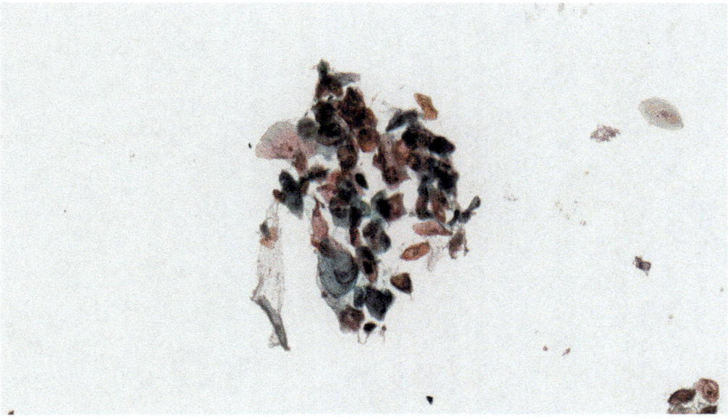

Fig. 7.3 Low grade dysplasia and koilocytosis in oral squamous cells as observed in liquid-based cytology (Papanicolaou stain- mag. ×200)

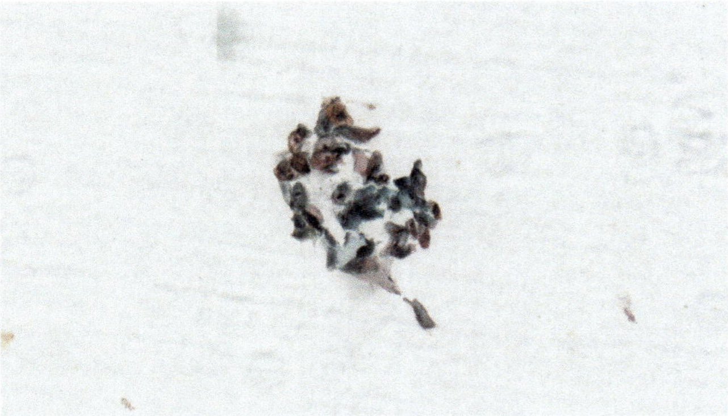

Fig. 7.4 Low grade dysplasia and koilocytosis in oral squamous cells as observed in liquid-based cytology (Papanicolaou stain- mag. ×200)

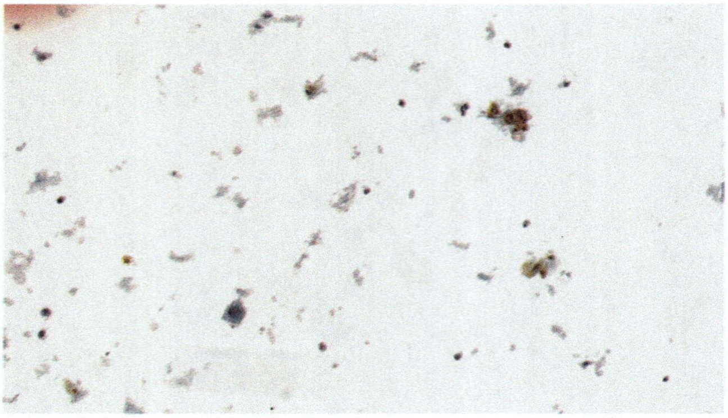

Fig. 7.5 High grade dysplasia in oral squamous cells as observed in liquid-based cytology (Papanicolaou stain- mag. ×200)

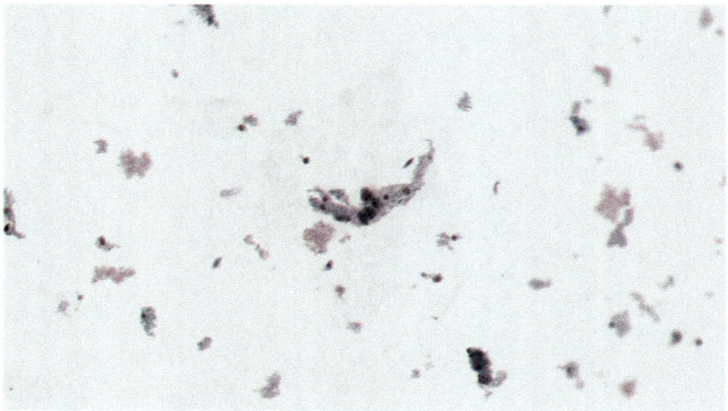

Fig. 7.6 High grade dysplasia in oral squamous cells as observed in liquid-based cytology (Papanicolaou stain- mag. ×200)

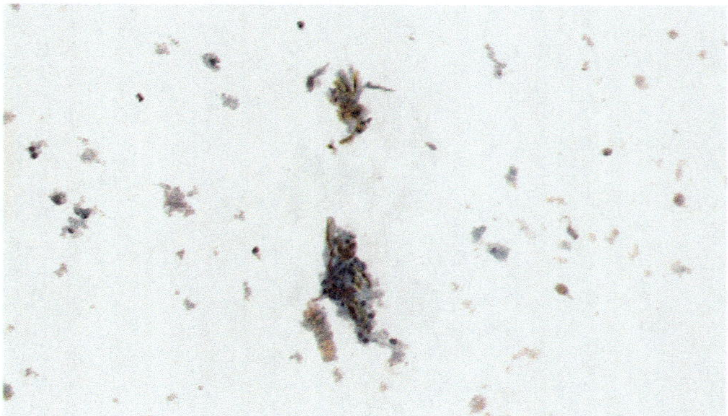

Fig. 7.7 Oral carcinoma cells as observed in liquid-based cytology (Papanicolaou stain- mag. ×200)

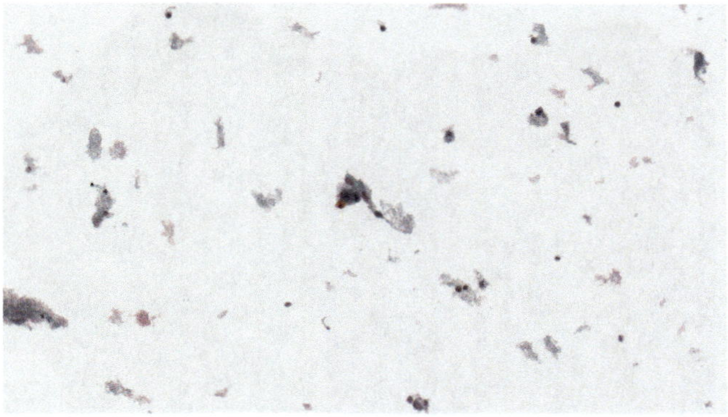

Fig. 7.8 Oral carcinoma cells as observed in liquid-based cytology (Papanicolaou stain- mag. ×200)

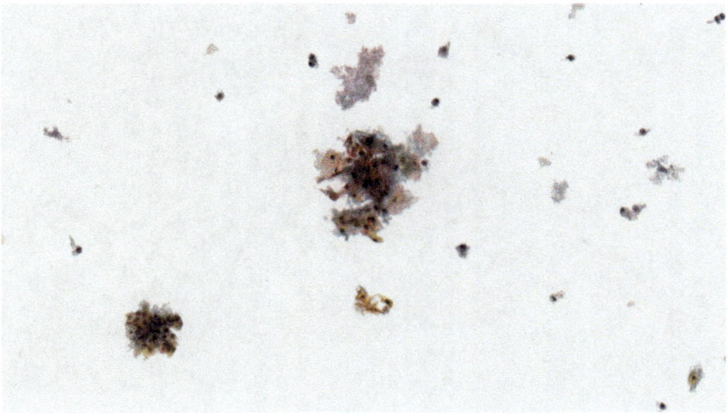

Fig. 7.9 Oral carcinoma cells as observed in liquid-based cytology (Papanicolaou stain- mag. ×200)

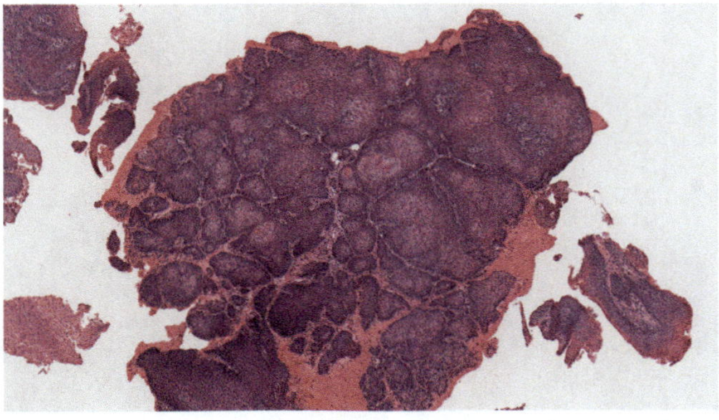

Fig. 7.10 Hyperkeratotic and acanthotic oral squamous epithelium as observed in microhistology (Hematoxylin-Eosin stain ×50)

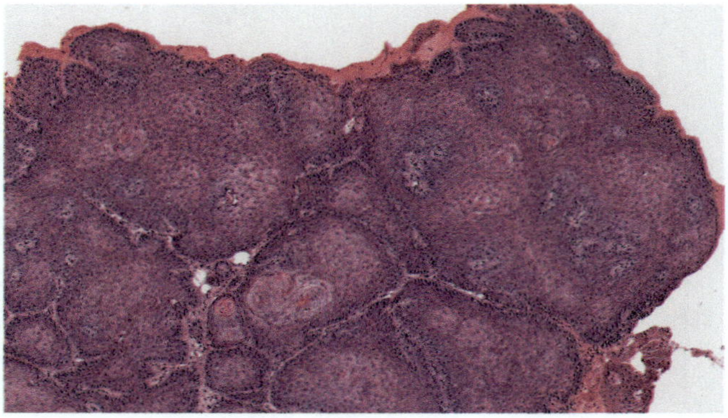

Fig. 7.11 Hyperkeratotic and acanthotic oral squamous epithelium as observed in microhistology

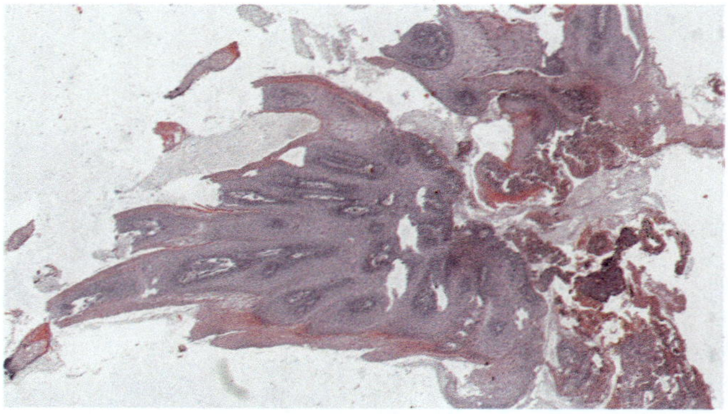

Fig. 7.12 Hyperkeratotic oral squamous papilloma as observed in microhistology (Hematoxylin-Eosin stain ×40)

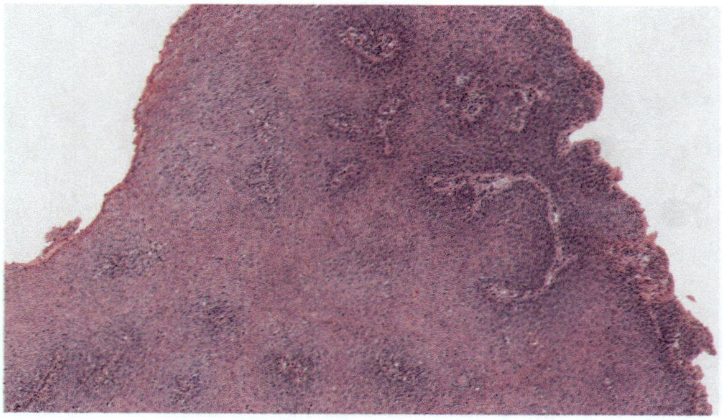

Fig. 7.13 Dysplastic (low grade) oral mucosa as observed in microhistology (Hematoxylin-Eosin stain ×100)

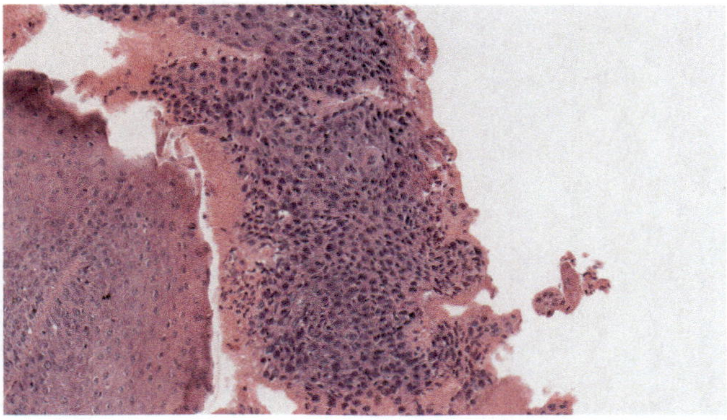

Fig. 7.14 Dysplastic (high grade) oral epithelium, close to normal mucosa, as observed in microhistology (Hematoxylin-Eosin stain ×200)

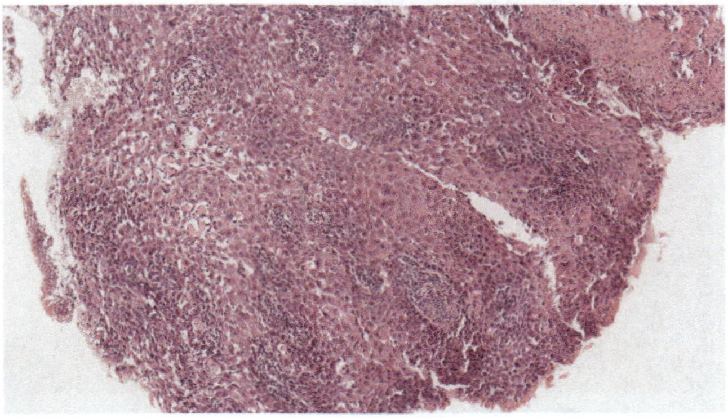

Fig. 7.15 Squamous oral carcinoma as observed in microhistology (Hematoxylin-Eosin stain ×100)

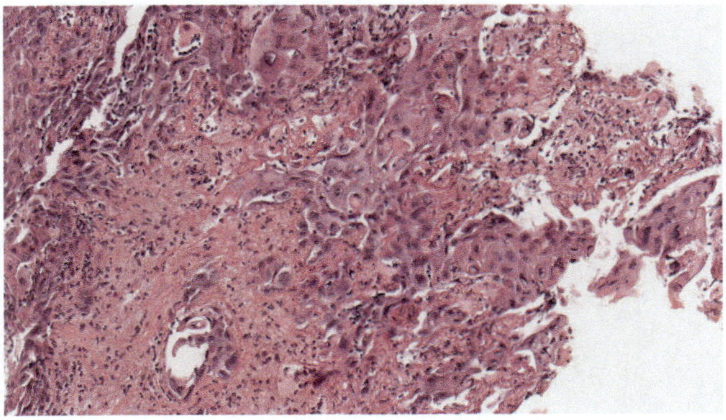

Fig. 7.16 Squamous oral carcinoma as observed in microhistology (Hematoxylin-Eosin stain ×200)

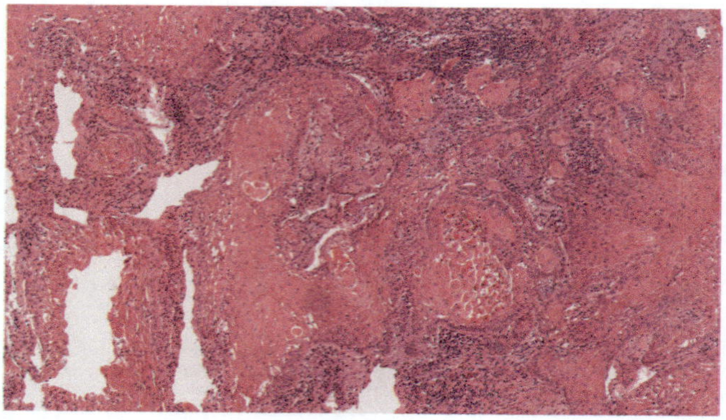

Fig. 7.17 Squamous oral carcinoma as observed in microhistology (Hematoxylin-Eosin stain ×100)

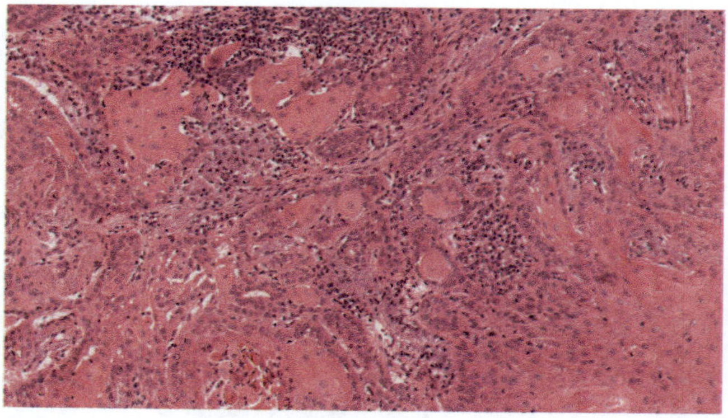

Fig. 7.18 Squamous oral carcinoma as observed in microhistology (Hematoxylin-Eosin stain ×200)

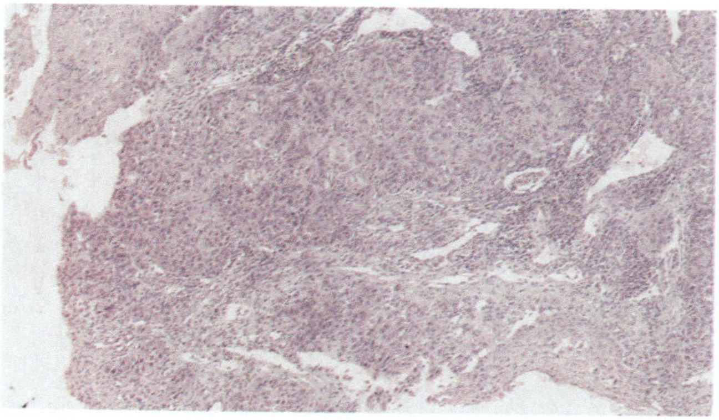

Fig. 7.19 Squamous oral carcinoma as observed in microhistology (Hematoxylin-Eosin stain ×100)

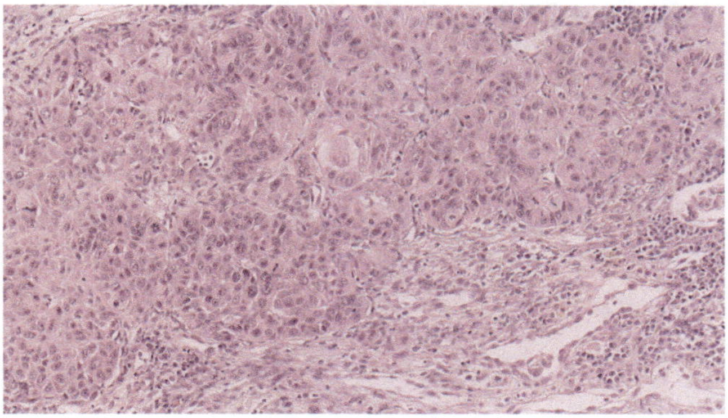

Fig. 7.20 Squamous oral carcinoma as observed in microhistology (Hematoxylin-Eosin stain ×200)

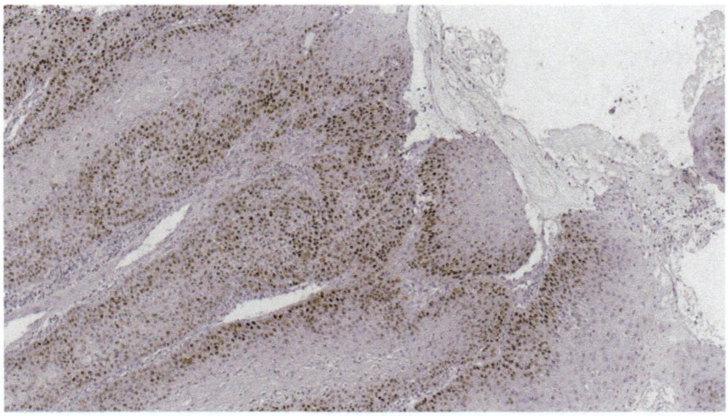

Fig. 7.21 p53 immunohistochemistry in squamous oral carcinoma as observed in microhistology (p53 ×100)

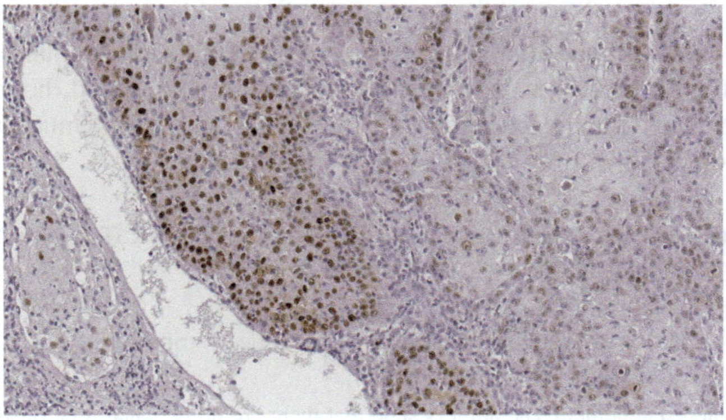

Fig. 7.22 p53 immunohistochemistry in squamous oral carcinoma as observed in microhistology (p53 ×200)

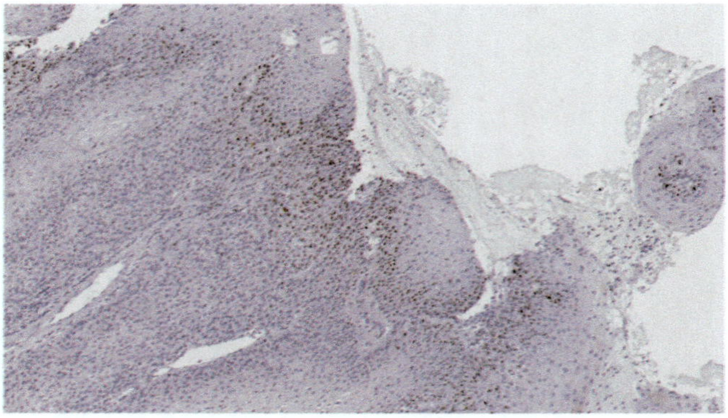

Fig. 7.23 Ki67 immunohistochemistry in squamous oral carcinoma as observed in microhistology (Ki67 ×100)

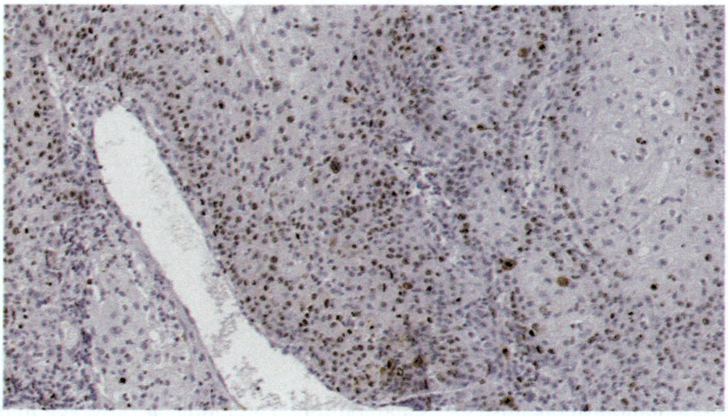

Fig. 7.24 Ki67 immunohistochemistry in squamous oral carcinoma as observed in microhistology (Ki67 ×200)

it is in the dentist's hands that most of the pre-neoplastic and neoplastic lesions are observed for the first time. The adoption of this strategy could, hopefully, make a contribution in reducing the percentage of late diagnosis in oral mucosal squamous cell carcinoma.

Acknowledgments This study has been supported in part by MURST ex-60% "*Università di Torino", Ricerca Finalizzata Regione Piemonte* and by a grant of the "*Compagnia di San Paolo-Programma Oncologia*", Turin, Italy.

The authors also thank Mrs. Barbara Wade for her linguistic contribution.

Conflict of interest statement The authors state that there are no personal relationships with other people or organizations that could have inappropriately influenced their work.

References

1. International Agency for Research on Cancer – World Health: The GLOBOCAN 2002 database.
2. Rosso S, Casella C, Crocetti E, Ferretti S, Guzzinati S. Survival of cancer patients in Italy in the nineties. Epidemiol Prev (Suppl) 2001; 25: 1–375.
3. Smeets SJ, Brakenhoff RH, Yistra B, van Wieringen WN, van der Wiel MA, Leemans CR, Braakhuis BJ. Genetic classification of oral and oropharyngeal carcinomas identifies subgroups with a different prognosis. Cell Oncol. 2009;31:291–300.
4. Mehanna H, Jones TM, Gregoire V, Ang KK. Oropharyngeal carcinoma related to human papilloma virus. BMJ. 2010;340:c1439.
5. La Vecchia C, Lucchini F, Negri E, Levi F. Trends in oral cancer mortality in Europe. Oral Oncol. 2004;40:433–9.
6. Sankaranarayanan R, Ramadas K, Thomas G, Muwonge R, Thara S, Mathew B, Rajan B, Trivandrum Oral Cancer Screening Study Group. Effect of screening on oral cancer mortality in Kerala, India: a cluster-randomised controlled trial. Lancet. 2005;365:1927–33.
7. Rethman MP, Cter W, Cohen EE, Epstein J, Evans CA, Flaitz CM, Graham FG, Hujoel PP, Kalmar JR, Koch WM, Lambert PM, Lingen MW, Oettmeier Jr BW, Patton LL, Perkins D, Reid BC, Sciubba JJ, Tomar SL, Wyatt Jr AD, Aravamudhan K, Frantsve-Hawley J, Cleveland JL, Meyer DM. Evidence-based clinical recommendations regarding screening for oral squamous cell carcinomas. J Am Dent Assoc. 2010;141:509–20.
8. Lingen MW, Kalmar JR, Karrison T, Speight PM. Critical evaluation of diagnostic aids for the detection of oral cancer. Oral Oncol. 2008;44:10–22.
9. Mehrotra R, Hullmann M, Smeets R, Reichert TE, Driemel O. Oral cytology revisited. J Oral Pathol Med. 2009;38:161–6.
10. Trullenque-Eriksson A, Munoz-Corcuera M, Campo-Trapero J, Cano-Sanchez J, Bascones-Martinez A. Analysis of new diagnostic methods in suspicious lesions of the oral mucosa. Med Oral Patol Oral Cir Bucal. 2009;14:E210–6.
11. Pérez-Sayansm M, Somoza-Martin JM, Barros-Angueira F, Reboiras-Lopez MD, Gandara-Vila P, Gandara Rey JM, Garcia-Garcia A. Exfoliative cytology for diagnosing oral cancer. Biotech Histochem. 2010;85:177–87.
12. Patton LL, Epstein JB, Kerr AR. Adjunctive techniques for oral cancer examination and lesion diagnosis. J Am Dent Assoc. 2008;139:896–905.
13. Pentenero M, Broccoletti R, Carbone M, Conrotto D, Gandolfo S. The prevalence of oral mucosal lesions in adults from the Turin area. Oral Dis. 2008;14:356–66.
14. Pentenero M, Carrozzo M, Pagano M, Galliano D, Broccoletti R, Scully C, Gandolfo S. Oral mucosal dysplastic lesions and early squamous carcinomas: underdiagnosis from incisional biopsy. Oral Dis. 2003;9:68–72.
15. Fedele S. Diagnostic aids in the screening of oral cancer. Head Neck Oncol. 2009;1:5–11.
16. Allegra SR, Broderick PA, Noama Corvese CT. Oral cytology: 7 year oral cytology screening programme in the state of Rhode Island. Analysis of 6,448 cases. Acta Cytol. 1973;17:42–8.
17. Parida G. Diagnostic cells in scrape cytology of squamous cell carcinoma. Acta Cytol. 2001;45:1085–6.
18. Navone R, Marsico A, Reale I, Pich A, Broccoletti R, Pentenero M, Gandolfo S. Usefulness of oral cytology on the diagnosis of oral squamous dysplasia and carcinoma. Minerva Stomatol. 2004;53:77–86.
19. Caruntu I-D, Scutariu MM, Dobrescu G. Computerized morphometric discrimination between normal and tumoral cells in oral smears. J Cell Mol Med. 2005;9:160–8.
20. Navone R, Burlo P, Pich A, Pentenero M, Broccoletti R, Marsico A, Gandolfo S. The impact of liquid-based cytology for the diagnosis of oral dysplasia and carcinoma. Cytopathology. 2007;18:356–60.
21. Delavarian Z, Mohtasham N, Mosannen-Mozafari P, Pakfetrat A, Shakeri MT, Ghafoorian-Maddah R. Evaluation of the diagnostic value of a modified liquid-based cytology using OralCDx® brush in early detection of oral potentially malignant lesions and oral cancer. Med Oral Patol Oral Cir Bucal. 2010;15(5):e671–6.

22. Kujan O, Desai M, Sargent A, Bailey A, Turner A, Sloan P. Potential applications of oral brush cytology with liquid-based technology: results from a cohort of normal human mucosa. Oral Oncol. 2006;42:810–8.
23. Hayama FH, Motta ACF, Silva APG, Migliari DA. Liquid-based preparations versus conventional cytology: specimen adequacy and diagnostic agreement in oral lesions. Med Oral Patol Oral Cir Bucal. 2005;10:115–22.
24. Mehrotra R, Mishra S, Singh M, Singh M. The efficacy of oral brush biopsy with computer-assisted analysis in identifying precancerous and cancerous lesions. Head Neck Oncol. 2011;3:39.
25. Marsico A, Demurtas A, Burlo P, Rostan L, Pentenero M, Gandolfo S, Navone R. Liquid-based diagnostic cytology of oral potentially malignant lesions (PML): DNA analysis with flow cytometry. 32nd European Congress of Cytology, Venice 1–3 October 2006.
26. Pentenero M, Giaretti W, Navone R, Demurtas A, Rostan I, Bertolusso G, Broccoletti R, Arduino PG, Malacarne D, Gandolfo S. DNA aneuploidy and dysplasia in oral potentially malignant disorders: association with cigarette smoking and site. Oral Oncol. 2009;45:887–90.
27. Donadini A, Maffei M, Cavallero A, Pentenero M, Malacarne D, Di Nallo E, Truini M, Navone R, Mereu P, Scala M, Santelli A, Gandolfo S, Giaretti W. Oral cancer genesis and progression: DNA near-diploid aneuplodization and endoreduplication by high resolution flow cytometry. Cell Oncol. 2010;32:373–83.
28. Pentenero M, Donadini A, Familiari U, Navone R, Di Nallo E, Castagnola P, Gandolfo S, Giaretti W. Chromosomal instability as assessed by high resolution DNA flow cytometry oral squamous cell carcinoma versus oral verrucous carcinoma. It J Maxillofac Surg 2011: 22 (1 Suppl 2): 60.
29. Tsui FL, Garnis C, Poh CF. A dynamic oral cancer field. Unraveling the underlying biology and its clinical implications. Am J Surg Pathol. 2009;33:1732–8.
30. Graveland AP, De Maaker M, Braakhuis BJM, De Bree R, Eerenstein SEJ, Bloemena E, Leemans CR, Brakenhoff RH. Molecular detection of minimal residual cancer in surgical margins of head and neck cancer patients. Cell Oncol. 2009;31:317–28.
31. Torres-Rendon A, Steward R, Craig GT, Wells M, Speight PM. DNA ploidy analysis by image cytometry helps to identify oral epithelial dysplasias with a high risk of malignant progression. Oral Oncol. 2009;45:468–73.
32. Navone R, Marsico A, Rostan I, Pentenero M, Gandolfo S. Exfoliative cytology and micro-histology of oral potentially malignant lesions (PMLs): an analysis of performance using a new sampling method. Cytopathology 2008; 19 (Suppl): 44.
33. Navone R, Pentenero M, Rostan I, Burlo P, Marsico A, Scully C, Gandolfo S. Oral potentially malignant lesions: first level micro-histological diagnosis from tissue fragments sampled in liquid-based diagnostic cytology. J Oral Pathol Med. 2008;37:358–63.
34. Navone R, D'Angelo G, Rostan I, Marsico A, Pentenero M, Tempia Valenta G, Gandolfo S. Oral microhistology: an innovative technique for a first level diagnosis in oral oncology for the practical odontostomatologist. It J Maxillofac Surg 2011; 22 (1 Suppl.2): 66.
35. Navone R, Pentenero M, Gandolfo S. Liquid-based cytology in oral cavity squamous cell cancer. Curr Opin Otolaryngol Head Neck Surg. 2011;19:77–81.
36. Cruz I, Napier SS, van der Waal I, Snijders PJF, Walboomers JMM, Lamey PJ, Cowan CG, Gregg TA, Maxwell P. Suprabasal p53 immunoexpression is strongly associated with high grade dysplasia and risk for malignant transformation in potentially malignant oral lesions from Northerrn Ireland. J Clin Pathol. 2002;55:98–104.
37. Angiero F, Berenzi A, Benetti A, Rossi E, Del Sordo R, Sidoni A, Stefani M, Dessy E. Expression of p16, p53 and Ki-67 proteins in the progression of epithelial dysplasia of the oral cavity. Anticancer Res. 2008;28:2535–9.
38. Takeda T, Sugihara K, Hirayama Y, Hirano M, Tanuma J-I, Semba I. Immunohistological evaluation of Ki-67, p63, CK19 and p53 expression in oral epithelial dysplasias. J Oral Pathol Med. 2006;35:369–75.
39. Tarakji B, Kujjan O, Nassani MZ. An immunohistochemical study of the distribution of p16 protein in oral mucosa in smokers, non-smokers and in frictional keratosis. Med Oral Patol Oral Cir Bucal. 2010;15(5):e681–4.

Chapter 8
The Role of Ploidy Analysis in Oral Cytology

Torsten W. Remmerbach

Cytogenetic Backgrounds

All types of tumors, even benign ones, may show numerical and structural chromosomal aberrations, which are not present in healthy or reactive cells [1].

During progression of the tumor, early detectable and cancer specific primary aberrations are followed by secondary and tertiary chromosomal changes. Primary aberrations are the first cytogenetic structural or numeric changes, which are detectable by the conventional light microscope. Only one or a few chromosomes are hit specifically and mainly persistent during tumor progression. These changes are type specific for distinct malignancies like Philadelphia chromosomes in chronic myeloid leukemia. Solid tumors mostly present deletions of chromosomes, leukemia, however, is largely characterized by translocations. These early chromosomal changes are followed by secondary aberrations and affect specific chromosomes on a regular base; this leads to worsening the prognosis of the patient's disease [2]. In contrast to the primary ones, secondary aberrations are detectable by quantification of the net effect of the cellular DNA content using image DNA cytometry [3]. Tertiary chromosomal aberrations are the result of genetic instability and may affect chromosomes at random.

In principle, the analysis of chromosomes is capable of qualifying cells to be malignant, independently by histological or cytological examination [2, 4]. Even earlier stages of malignancy without clinical symptoms and the malignant potential may be determined by chromosomal analysis. But these complex cytogenetic techniques are not available for all types of tissues due to the lack of sufficient cell culture capability to transfer the cells into the M-phase. Additionally they are elaborate and time consuming.

T.W. Remmerbach (✉)
Oral Medicine Unit, Department of Oral, Maxillofacial and Facial Plastic Surgery, University of Leipzig, Liebigstr. 10-14 (Haus 1), 04103 Leipzig, Germany
e-mail: torsten.remmerbach@uniklinik-leipzig.de

R. Mehrotra (ed.), *Oral Cytology: A Concise Guide*, DOI 10.1007/978-1-4614-5221-8_8,

Feulgen Staining

The DNA content cannot be measured directly by cytometry. After quantitative DNA staining, the nuclear Integrated Optical Density (IOD) is the cytometric equivalent of its DNA content. Subsequently all specimens must be destained and additionally Feulgen stained in a temperature-controlled staining machine with Schiff's reagent [5].

The Feulgen staining procedure is a well-established and frequently documented procedure for quantitative DNA staining [5]. The principle of this staining process is based on two steps: In the first step the double stranded DNA must be split off the purine bases, therefore it must be hydrolyzed by a strong acid, like 5 M HCl for 55 min. This results in an apurinic acid that shows aldehyde groups at the former positions of the purine base on the DNA strand. The destaining of prestained slides after Papanicolaou staining is made in this step as well.

Secondly, the Schiff base, like basic parafuchsin, binds stoichiometrically to the aldehyde groups of the DNA and this results in a reddish colored nucleus with an absorption maximum of 570 nm.

Studies have shown that the staining intensity depends strictly on the temperature of the DNA hydrolysis in 5 M HCl of the DNA; the optimum hydrolysis temperature is 27°C and even changes of 0.5°C affect the measurement of the IOD significantly [5–7]. For application in routine diagnostic procedures, the staining should be standardized to assure reliable and reproducible results.

The DNA cytometry is a quantitative measurement and thus all cells on the glass slide must be stained in a similar way; reference cells on the identical slide have to be taken as an internal standard. Differences of the staining intensity occurring within the same slide may lead to incorrect calibration and thus to false ploidy values. Therefore the application of an automated staining machine is strictly recommended. For example the commercially available Shandon Varistain 24 staining machine can be run automatically and (flow-through) cuvettes are 24 h temperature controlled, if necessary [5]. The storage must be in the dark to avoid fading effects of the slides. The Feulgen stained slides can be re-stained to PAP easily for conventional re-evaluation.

Preparation of Specimens

The slides of alcohol-fixed, Papanicolaou-stained, routine smears from mucosal brushings should be evaluated according to the published guidelines for extra genital cytology [8]. This is necessary to define normal, doubtful, suspicious or unequivocal tumor cells on the slide. The precondition for a proper DNA analysis is the marking/circling of these cells with a felt pen on the glass slide prior to Feulgen staining. This procedure is followed by photocopying the slides to assure the remarking after removal of the cover slip. Afterwards cover slips should be removed carefully after xylol treatment. The time depends on the time of archiving the specimens.

Never use force for removal, you may dislodge cells from the slide. After staining the areas of interests must be re-marked on the slides using the photocopies.

After rehydration in decreasing ethanol concentrations and refixation in buffered 10% formalin, 5 N HCL for acid hydrolysis was applied at 27°C for 55 min, followed by staining in Schiff's reagent (Merck, Darmstadt, Germany) for another hour, followed by rinsing in SO_2-water to remove surplus dye from cell nuclei and cytoplasm. Dehydration at increasing ethanol concentrations is followed [9]. The slides must then be covered with Entellan (Merck, Darmstadt, Germany) and stored in the dark.

DNA-Image Cytometry/DNA-Measurements

The aim of diagnostic DNA cytometry is to identify DNA stem lines outside the euploid regions as abnormal (or aneuploid) at a defined statistic level of significance. The numerical and/or structural chromosomal aberrations are the biological basis for DNA-Image cytometry. The quantitation of nuclear DNA requires a rescaling of the measured Integrated Optical Density (IOD) values by comparison with those from cells with known DNA content. Therefore the DNA content is expressed in a "c" scale in which 1c is half the mean nuclear DNA content of cells from a normal (non-pathological) diploid population in G0/G1 cell cycle phase. A DNA-stem line was defined as a frequency peak in a histogram accompanied by values at its two-fold DNA-content. It was defined interactively when the DNA-histograms were displayed on the screen by marking its minimum and maximum [9–11] (Fig. 8.1).

The photometric analysis of the integrated optical density was performed by the QUIC-DNA system (TriPath, Burlington, NC, USA) in combination with a conventional light microscope Axioplan 2 (Zeiss, Jena, Germany) with the objectives 40/0,75; 20/0,40; 10/0,25 and 4/0,10. To reduce stray light, the Köhler measurement was performed and an interference filter 570 nm ± 10 nm was used. The TriPath system was interfaced with a 486 IBM-compatible personal computer with a frame grabber card (Matrox electronics, Munich, Germany) using a TV camera with 572 lines (VarioVam CCIR, PCO Computer Optics, Kehlheim, Germany) with a magnification of factor 1.6. Segmentation was performed automatically on individual nuclei by gray level thresholding, taking the local background into consideration for each nucleus. The glare- and diffraction errors were corrected by software as proposed by Kindermann and Hilgers [12]. The data were interpreted using the analysis software of the system.

The normal 2c reference value was established by measuring 30 cytologically normal epithelial cells or lymphocytes on each slide as an internal reference (mean values of integrated optical densities (IOD)). CVs (=coefficient of variation) of reference cells must be below 5%. No correction factor was applied. If present, three hundred atypical epithelial or carcinoma cells per specimen were measured interactively at random. The performance of the system meets the standards of the European Society for Analytical Cellular Pathology (ESACP) task force on standardization of diagnostic DNA-image cytometry [9–11, 13].

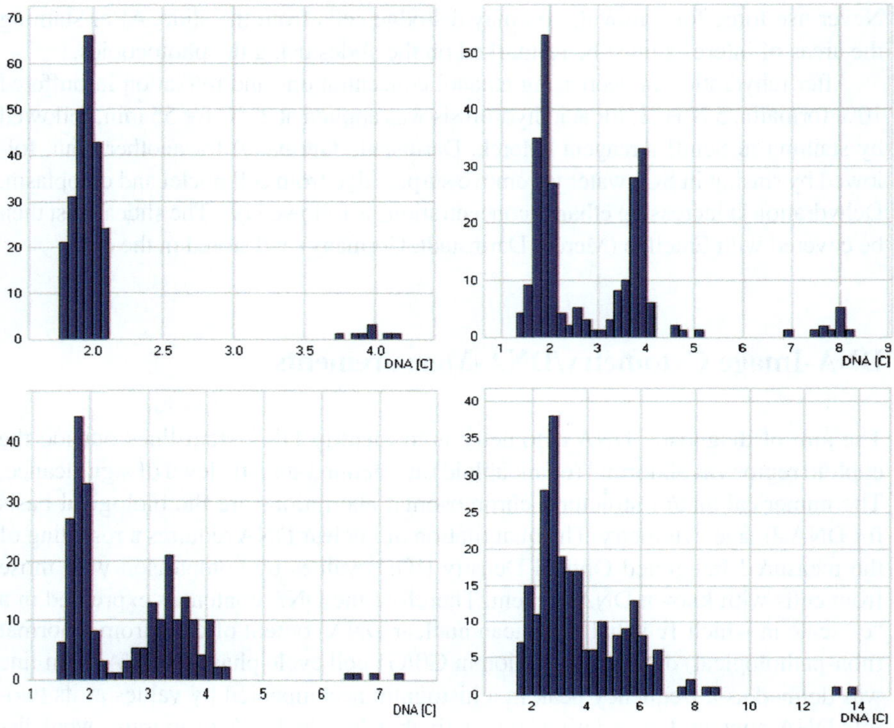

Fig. 8.1 *Top left*: 2. DNA-histogram of a smear from a histologically proven hyperkeratosis without dysplasia, showing number of cells measured (n) and their corresponding DNA-content (c) and a (*normal*) diploid stem line at 2.0c. *Top right*: DNA-histogram of a smear from a Lichen planus (erosive), showing (euploid) polyploid stem lines at 2.0c and 4.0c. *Bottom left*: DNA-histogram of a smear from a squamous cell carcinoma of the tongue. An abnormal stem line at 1.7c and 3.5 can be detected as an aspect of DNA-aneuploidy. *Bottom right*: DNA-histogram of a smear from a squamous cell carcinoma of the alveolar ridge. Abnormal stem lines are shown, additionally, four cells with a DNA-content greater than 9c (9cEE) can be detected as another aspect of DNA-aneuploidy

Aspects of DNA-aneuploidy according to the Consensus reports of the European Society for Analytical and Cellular Pathology (1995, 1998, 2001) are as follows:

1. In comparison to the normal proliferating cell population (G0/G1-phase-fraction) to the analyzing cell population show an abnormal stem line with the most frequent value, i.e. the mean value of the histogram class containing the highest number of nuclei, which differs at least at 10% from those of normal (resting, proliferating, or polyploidizing) cell populations. The DNA index of the stem line must be <0.90>1.10 or <1.80>2/20 or <3.60>4.40.
2. Abnormal cells with a DNA content higher than 9c are present. Often called 9c exceeding events, are those cells having nuclear DNA content higher than the duplication or quadruplication region of a normal G0/G1 phase population, i.e. not belonging to G2/M phase fractions (cells >9c occurred (9c exceeding events [9cEE])) [14].

The quantity of nuclear DNA may be changed by the following mechanisms: replication, polyploidization, gain or deletion. Each affects the size or the number of chromatids. Furthermore viral infections may change the nuclear DNA content detectable by image cytometry. Among others, the unspecific effects of cytostatic or radiation therapy, vitamin B_{12} deficiency, apoptosis, autolysis and necrosis on nuclear DNA content play also a role [1, 15–19].

Clinical Impact of DNA-Image Cytometry for Oral Cancer Diagnosis

Primary Oral Squamous Cell Carcinomas

Our study group [20] has shown that specimens from healthy mucosa did not show any signs of aneuploidy according to the current Consensus reports of the ESACP. In a preliminary study, we have investigated 100 brush biopsies of benign, reactive or inflamed oral lesions and the modal value of the DNA stem line was nearly 2c (MV 2.01c; SD ±0.06). The correlation coefficient was 3.85%; 44 cases showed cells with cells >5c (Table 8.1). In a second step we investigated 100 brush biopsies from clinically unequivocal and histologically proven OSCCs: All hundred cases of cancer fulfilled the criteria for DNA aneuploidy. Thus all the cancer specimens showed one, two or both criteria of aneuploidy. Table 8.2 shows the incidence of the different criteria of aneuploidy. The presence of abnormal stemlines is seen in 9% of all aneuploid cases; 9c exceeding events (9cEE) were seen in 32% in aneuploid specimens. The occurrence of both, 9cEE and abnormal stemlines were seen in 59% of all cases.

The results of these pilot studies suggested strongly that aneuploidy detection may be a useful marker for discrimination of clinically doubtful lesions and may help to clarify their biological nature.

Additionally, we investigated 543 cases of brush biopsies from different doubtful lesions of the oral cavity in daily routine practice. In 53 cases, the DNA measurement was not possible due to technical limitations: (a) insufficient numbers of cells for proper analysis and (b) massive overlapping of cells and or nucleoli.

If present, 300 atypical epithelial or carcinoma cells per specimen were measured interactively, at random. Otherwise, only the available cells were measured: one (suspicious) case with 48 cells (=insufficient for DNA-cytometry); two cases with 51–100 measurable cells; four cases with 101–150 cells; six cases with 151–200 cells; seven cases with 201–250 cells; seven cases with 251–300 cells and all other cases with more than 300 cells. No stem line interpretation of DNA-aneuploidy was performed if less than 50 abnormal or atypical cells were contained. All inconspicuous cases (“tumor cell negative”) were measured using at least 30 reference cells and 300 analysis cells.

Overall, 304 cases showed no criteria of DNA aneuploidy. However 184 cases showed DNA aneuploidy, three cancer cases showed none of the criteria and were evaluated as non-aneuploid. The combination of abnormal stem line and cells

Table 8.1 Frequency of fulfilled criteria of DNA-aneuploidy in histologically proven benign lesions and cytological as "tumor cell negative" evaluated oral lesions ($n=100$)

Aspects of DNA-aneuploidy	[n]	%
Normal stemline [1,8 < c > 2,2] ˣ x=1 or 2 or 3	**100**	**100.0**
Atypical stemline [1,8 > c < 2,2] ˣ x=1 or 2 or 3		
1	**0**	**0**
2		
> 2		
Cells > 9cEE		
1 to 3		
4 to 10		
> 10		
Abnormal stemline and cells > 9cEE	**0**	**0**
SUM		**100.0**

Table 8.2 Frequency of fulfilled criteria of DNA-aneuploidy in histologically proven squamous cell carcinomas of the oral cavity and cytologically as "tumor cell positive" evaluated oral lesions ($n=100$)

Aspects of DNA-aneuploidy	[n]	%
Normal stemline [1,8 < c > 2,2] ˣ x=1,2,3	0	0
Atypical stemline [1,8 > c < 2,2] ˣ x=1,2,3		
1	5	5.0
2	3	3.0
> 2	1	1.0
Cells > 9cEE		
1 to 3	16	16.0
4 to 10	9	9.0
> 10	7	7.0
Abnormal stemline and cells > 9cEE	39	39.0
SUM	100	100.0

>9cEE was the major criteria of aneuploidy (60%), followed by 9cEE alone (29%) and abnormal stem lines with 11%. These data were in accordance with the pilot study mentioned above. The diagnostic accuracy is summarized as follows: The sensitivity was 98.4%, the specificity was 99.34%. The positive predictive value was 98.92% and the negative predictive value 99.01%. (For details see Table 8.3).

Lip Cancer

We investigated 27 cases of suspicious lesions of the lip, of which, 25 cases were technically sufficient for DNA analysis. All benign cases from lesions of the lip showed euploidy. In 16 cases of proven cancer, 11 cases fulfilled the aspects of

Table 8.3 Frequency of fulfilled criteria of DNA-aneuploidy in histologically proven squamous cell carcinomas of the oral cavity and cytologically as "tumor cell positive" evaluated oral lesions ($n=187$)

Aspects of DNA-aneuploidy	Conventional cytology[a]								
	Positive	%	sus	%	dft	%	Negative	Sum	%
Normal stemline [1,8 < c < 2,2]^{x} x=1,2,3			1				2	3	1.6
Atypical stemline [1,8 > c > 2,2]^{x} x=1,2,3	**13**	**8.55**	**4**	**17.4**	**4**	**44.4**		**21**	**11.2**
1	*6*		*3*		*4*				
2	*5*								
> 2	*2*		*1*						
Cells > 9cEE	**44**	**28.95**	**8**	**34.8**	**2**	**22.2**		**54**	**28.9**
1 to 3	*22*		*4*		*1*				
4 to 10	*13*		*4*		*1*				
> 10	*9*								
Abnormal stemline and **cells > 9cEE**	**95**	**62.50**	**11**	**47.8**	**3**	**33.3**		**109**	**58.3**
Aspects of aneuploidy	**152**		**23**		**9**		**0**	**184**	
SUM	**152**		**24**		**9**		**2**	**187**	**100.0**

[a] "tumor cell negative" (negative); "doubtful" (dft); "suspicious for tumor cells" (sus); "tumor cell positive" (positive)

aneuploidy, five patients showed normal euploid stem line. But the conventional cytological revaluation showed no evidence of cancer cells on these slides. Nevertheless the sensitivity of DNA-aneuploidy was 67% only; the specificity was 100%. The main criterion for aneuploidy was the presence of abnormal stem lines in 10% of all cases. Abnormal stem lines including 9c exceeding events were seen in 45% of the cases, followed by 9cEEs as a single marker in 45% of all measured cases (Table 8.4). Major limitations in these cases were the small number of cells, harvested with the nylon based cell collector. Even the maceration of the lips with physiologic salt solution prior to sampling did not increase the number of harvested cells significantly [20].

Reliability

To investigate the reliability of image DNA-cytometry, we calculated the intra-observer reliability; it is the variation in measurements taken by a single person on the same item and under the same conditions. In a second step, we determined the inter-observer reliability; this means the variation in measurements when taken by different persons but with the same method or instruments.

Table 8.4 Frequency of fulfilled criteria of DNA-aneuploidy in histologically proven squamous cell carcinomas of the lips and cytologically as "tumor cell positive" evaluated oral lesions ($n=16$)

Aspects of DNA-aneuploidy	Conventional cytology[a] Positive	%	sus	%	dft	%	Negative	Sum	%
Normal stemline [1,8 < c < 2,2] [x] x=1,2,3							5	5	31.25
Atypical stemline [1,8 > c > 2,2] [x] x=1,2,3	0	0.0	0	0.0	0	0.0	1	1	6.25
1							*1*		
2									
> 2									
Cells > 9cEE	3	1.97	1	4.3	1	11.1	0	5	31.25
1 to 3	*1*		*1*		*1*				
4 to 10	*1*								
> 10									
Abnormal stemline and **cells > 9cEE**	4	2.63	0	0.0	1	11.1	0	5	31.25
Aspects of Aneuploidy	7		1		2		6	11	
SUM	**7**		**1**		**2**		**6**	**16**	**100.0**

[a] "tumor cell negative" (negative); "doubtful" (dft); "suspicious for tumor cells" (sus); "tumor cell positive" (positive)

Therefore, we chose 137 specimens of oral brush biopsies out of 1,000 archived cases at random. The diagnoses were: 65 (47.45%) oral squamous cell carcinomas, thereof 55 (84.62%) primary carcinomas, 3 (4.62%) cases of recurrent cancer, 2 (3.08%) cases of secondary tumor and 5 (7.68%) cases of lip cancer. Out of 137 cases, 72 (52.55%) specimens came from clinically proven benign lesions.

All slides were independently analyzed by two observers to evaluate interobserver reliability of diagnosis of 137 cases; 2 month later identical specimens were re-evaluated by the same two observers to assess intraobserver reliability. The STATA program and Cohen's Kappa statistics were used to assess reliability. The calculation showed an (almost) perfect inter- and intraobserver ($k=0.99$) reliability according to Landis and Koch.

Laser Scanning Cytometry

The Laser scanning cytometry is a static cytometric DNA analysis that allows the measurement of fluorescent parameters of cells. It is a further development of the conventional flow cytometry, whereas the method combines the advantages of flow

Table 8.5 Overview of frequently used fluorochromes with optimal excitation wavelength, including of possible excitation by the LSC, emission maxima of fluorochromes and spectral borders of respective filters

Fluorochrome	Optimal excitation (nm)	Used excitation (nm)	Emission (nm)	Spectral borders of filters (nm)
FITC (Fluroreszeinthiocyanate)	495	488	519	515–545
R-PE (R-Phycoerythrine)	480 546 565	488	578	565–595
PI (Propidiumjodide)	535	488	617	611–639
APC (Allophycocyanine)	651 633	633 635	660	650 LP

and static image cytometry. The detected cell features are enlarged on the screen and multiple screen shots are taken for documentation purposes [21–25].

We have adapted Gerstner's assays [26, 27] for the fluorescent staining of different cytokeratins of oral keratinocytes with antibodies (Dako Cytomation, Hamburg, Germany) [20]. The clone MNF 116 for the cytokeratins 5, 6, 8, 17 and 19 was used. Due to the fact that not all squamous cells from carcinomas were stained; it seems likely that during carcinogenesis, epitopes were lost on the surface of the respective cells [27]. Therefore, we broadened the spectrum by using Clone beta E12, AE and AE3 (Dako Cytomation, Hamburg, Germany) to detect cytokeratin 1, 2, 3, 4, 5, 6, 8, 10, 14, 15, 16 and 19. The antibody was linked to streptavidin conjugated allophycocyanine (ACP). For details see Table 8.5.

The analysis was done by interpretation of the position of the stem line and the occurrence of 5cEE and 9cEE additionally [28].

We had evaluated 44 patients, including 22 oral squamous cell carcinomas. The sensitivity was 95.5%, the specificity 81.8%; the negative and positive predictive values were 84.0% and 94.7% respectively (Figs. 8.2–8.4). Gerstner and co-worker investigated 49 laryngeal lesions using cotton swabs and determined aneuploidy by stem line interpretation with the same laboratory setup: They achieved a sensitivity of 83% and a specificity of 93%, the negative predictive value was 67, the positive predictive value was around 88% [28].

Comparison of DNA-Image Cytometry Versus Laser Scanning Cytometry

All samples described in the previous chapter were re-stained and investigated by LSC and ICM as well. Out of 44 samples, one sample was technically insufficient for image cytometry due to significant cell loss by rigid removal of the cover slip. All 21 histograms of histologically proven cancer show aneuploidy and but none of

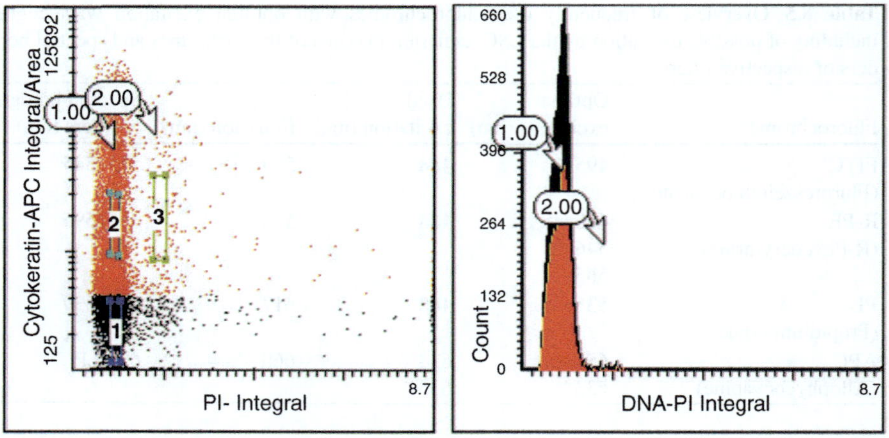

Fig. 8.2 *Left*: Dot plots of measured cell features. DNA-content (*x*-axis, linear) is plotted vs. APC-fluorescence per area (*y*-axis, logarithmic) (5% cut-off is set in the control sample–not shown). Three populations were definable: regions 1 and 3 (cytokeratin positive) and 2 (no cytokeratin ≈ lymphocytes ≈ internal reference). *Right*: The cells of region 1 showed a stem line with a DNA Index (DI) 1,0 and in region 2 showed a stem line with a DNA Index of 2

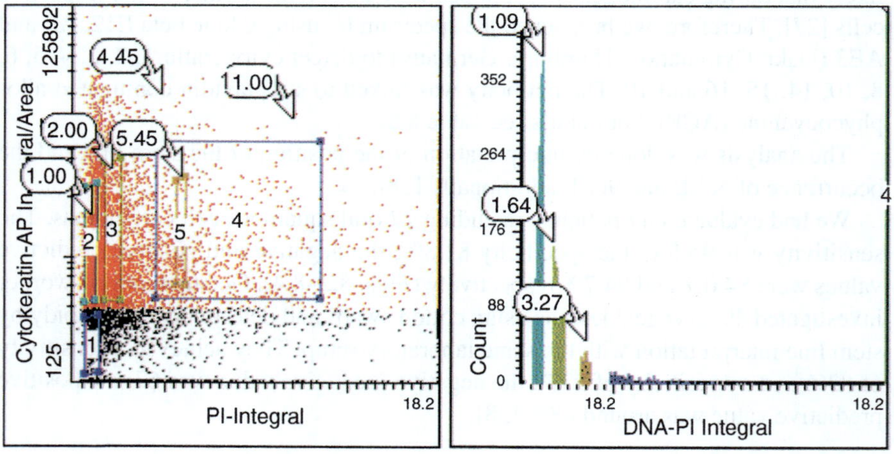

Fig. 8.3 A brush biopsy from a tongue carcinoma (pT3pN1cM0) was prepared according to the protocol (total cell count of the positive sample: 8,327). The set-up of the figure and acquisition of micrographs is equivalent to Fig. 8.1. The marked changes from normal cytokeratin-positive epithelium (DI = 1.09) to aneuploid carcinoma (DI = 1.64 and 3.27) are clearly visible. There are also cells with polyploid DNA content (DI > 5.0)

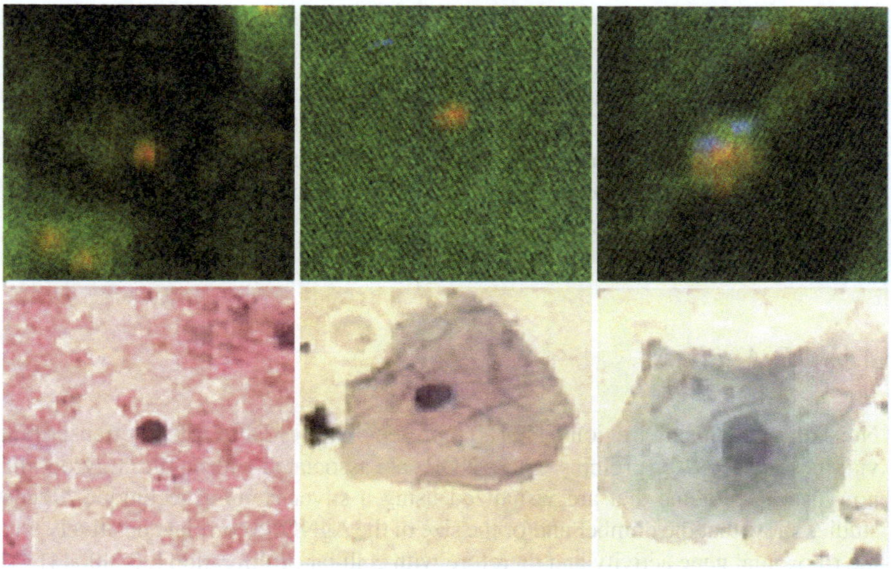

Fig. 8.4 Interpretation of LSC data: Brush biopsy (benign) was analyzed by LSC: pseudocolored images were taken by rescanning single cells (*upper lines*). Then, slides were stained with PAP, identical cells were relocalized, and images were taken (*lower lines*). Analysis and imaging were performed with the ×20 objective. (Note: Because of different optical pathways, corresponding images are symmetrical to their center)

the benign lesions: the combination of abnormal stem line and cells >9c were shown in 48% of all cases, abnormal stem lines in 42% and 9cEE in 10%. Thus the sensitivity and specificity were 100%.

The regression analysis (Pearson product–moment correlation coefficient) revealed 0.87 in comparison of both techniques. The major problem for the validity of the LSC was the stringent re-localisation after re-staining according to PAP to verify 9cEEs to reduce false negative results. This procedure extended the evaluation time up to 2–3 h per case [20].

Multi-modal Cell Analysis

The aim of this clinical study was to apply a novel approach to improve diagnostic accuracy by sequential analysis of cellular characteristics in the same smear using Multimodal Cell Analysis (MMCA) [29, 30]. We applied the MMCA process to smears from oral brush biopsies, combining conventional cytology with the more quantifiable DNA content, followed by Argyrophilic Nucleolar Organizing Regions (AgNOR) count, to identify early malignant transformation [31]. Recent studies have shown that the number and/or size of AgNORs correlate with the ribosomal gene activity and therefore with cellular proliferation and consequent malignant potential [32–36].

DNA-Measurements

The performance of our system, that is based on a Leica DMLA automated microscope, meets the standards of the European Society for Analytical Cellular Pathology (ESACP) task force on standardization of diagnostic DNA-Image cytometry [9, 10, 37].

Details of software algorithms for precise scene matching, re-localization and registration have been described in detail elsewhere [29, 38, 39].

AgNOR-Analysis

Nucleolar Organising Regions (NORs) represent loops of DNA actively transcribing via ribosomal RNA to proteins. These NORs are associated with acidic, argyrophilic, non-histone proteins that are visualized using a silver staining technique. Recent studies show that the number and/or the size of the AgNORs correlate positively with the ribosomal gene activity and therefore with cellular proliferation [33, 40–44].

Silver staining was performed according to the one step method by Ploton et al. [35] and Crocker et al. [45] with modifications [46]. Manual AgNOR counting was performed on 100 normal cells and abnormal squamous cells for each cytological smear. The mean number of AgNORs per nucleus as clusters, satellites, clusters and satellites together were considered.

All information gathered from different stains and evaluated by different methods of analysis contribute to the identification and characterization of cancerous or even precancerous cells.

In our oral cancer study the MMCA [31] process was operated as a stepwise process, as described previously. First, the operator selects representative regions on the stained slides containing atypical or abnormal cells. Images are immediately digitized and stored together with their coordinates. The slides are then de-stained and re-stained by the Feulgen method. The newly stained and covered slides are then placed back onto the microscope stage where the previously recorded coordinates stored in the database automatically reposition the slide to the regions of interest digitized before. Finally all cases received a third stain with silver nitrate to demonstrate AgNOR-dots. As before, a digital registration was performed on the digitized regions of interest. The results were appended to the feature set of the individual cells.

All 25 cytologically tumor negative specimens were DNA-non-euploid. 4/20 squamous cell carcinomas revealed an atypical DNA-stem line alone, 5/20 abnormal cells >9c alone and 9/20 both aspects of DNA-aneuploidy.

Sensitivity of DNA-aneuploidy on oral smears for the detection of cancer cells thus was 95%, specificity for the detection of benign lesions 100%, positive predictive value 100% and negative predictive value 96.4%.

AgNOR-analysis reached a sensitivity of 100% for the diagnosis of malignant cells, specificity of 100% for benign cells, whereas the cut-off level was determined by 5.09 AgNORs per nucleus, as described previously [46]. The negative predictive value reached 100% and the positive predictive value 100%.

The sequential application of different methods (e.g. DNA-cytometry, AgNOR-analysis) increased the sensitivity and specificity of our cytological diagnosis from 90% to 100%. Due to the hierarchical or cascaded approach of MMCA, a measurement of uncertain specimens is terminated at a certain stage, when a definitive cancer diagnosis is confirmed through additional information e.g. the presence of DNA-aneuploidy [31].

Conclusion

The prevalence of DNA aneuploidy is very high in oral cell carcinoma, on the contrary, in benign lesions it is nearly zero. Thus, as an independent marker, aneuploidy serves as a valid and reliable indicator for the identification of neoplasms of the oral cavity. The additional evaluation of conventional cytological specimens from brush biopsies by image cytometry improved the diagnostic accuracy of pathologist's daily routine. DNA-Image cytometry is well established and current studies support our results for specimens of oral brush biopsies [47–50].

References

1. Sandberg A. The chromosomes in human cancer and leukemia. Amsterdam, New York: Oxford Elsevier; 1990.
2. Heim S, Mitelman F. Cancer cytogenetics. New York: Alan R Liss, Inc; 1987. p. 239–40.
3. Böcking A, Wied GL, Keebler CM, et al. DNA measurements. When and Why? Compendium on quality assurance, proficiency testing, and workload limitations. Chicago, IL; 1995. p. 170–88.
4. Hansteen IL, Hilt B, Lien JT, Skaug V, Haugen A. Karyotypic changes in the preclinical and subsequent stages of malignant mesothelioma: a case report. Cancer Genet Cytogenet. 1993;70(2):94–8.
5. Chatelain R, Willms A, Biesterfeld S, Auffermann W, Böcking A. Automated Feulgen staining with a temperature-controlled staining machine. Anal Quant Cytol Histol. 1989;11(3):211–7.
6. Böcking A, Striepecke E, Auer H, et al. Static DNA-cytometry. Biological background, technique and diagnostic interpretation. Tutorials of Cytology. Chicago, IL; 1994. p. 107–128.
7. Nguyen VQ, Grote HJ, Pomjanski N, Knops K, Böcking A. Interobserver reproducibility of DNA-image-cytometry in ASCUS or higher cervical cytology. Cell Oncol. 2004;26(3):143–50.
8. Böcking A, Freudenberg N. Standardisierte Befunderstellung in der extragenitalen Zytologie. Pathologe. 1998;19:235–6.
9. Haroske G, Baak JP, Danielsen H, et al. Fourth updated ESACP consensus report on diagnostic DNA image cytometry. Anal Cell Pathol. 2001;23(2):89–95.
10. Böcking A, Giroud F, Reith A. Consensus report of the ESACP task force on standardization of diagnostic DNA image cytometry. European Society for Analytical Cellular Pathology. AnalCell Pathol. 1995;8(1):67–74.

11. Giroud F, Haroske G, Reith A, Böcking A. 1997 ESACP consensus report on diagnostic DNA image cytometry. Part II: specific recommendations for quality assurance. European Society for Analytical Cellular Pathology. Anal Cell Pathol. 1998;17(4):201–8.
12. Kindermann D, Hilgers CH. Glare-correction in DNA image cytometry. Anal Cell Pathol. 1994;6(2):165–80.
13. Haroske G, Meyer W, Oberholzer M, Böcking A, Kunze KD. Competence on demand in DNA image cytometry. Pathol Res Pract. 2000;196(5):285–91.
14. Chatelain R, Schunck T, Schindler EM, Schindler AE, Böcking A. Diagnosis of prospective malignancy in koilocytic dysplasias of the cervix with DNA cytometry. J Reprod Med. 1989;34(8):505–10.
15. Biesterfeld S, Fuzesi L, Härle F, Böcking A. DNA-cytometric detection of euploid polyploidization in oral lichen ruber planus. Anal Quant Cytol Histol. 1991;13(1):7–10.
16. Biesterfeld S, Gerres K, Fischer-Wein G, Böcking A. Polyploidy in non-neoplastic tissues. J Clin Pathol. 1994;47(1):38–42.
17. Böhm N, Sprenger E, Schluter G, Sandritter W. Proportionalitätsfehler bei der Feulgen-Hydrolyse. Histochemie. 1968;15:194–203.
18. Stenkvist B, Strande G. Entropy as an algorithm for the statistical description of DNA cytometric data obtained by image analysis microscopy. Anal Cell Pathol. 1990;2(3):159–65.
19. Stenkvist B, Olding-Stenkvist E. Cytological and DNA characteristics of hyperplasia/inflammation and cancer of the prostate. Eur J Cancer. 1990;26(3):261–7.
20. Remmerbach: Evaluation der zytologischen Diagnostik und adjuvanter Methoden an Präparaten oraler Bürstenbiopsien zur Sekundärprävention von Lippen- und Oropharynxkarzinomen. Leipzig: Univ., Habil.-Schrift; 2006.
21. Kamentsky LA, Kamentsky LD. Microscope-based multiparameter laser scanning cytometer yielding data comparable to flow cytometry data. Cytometry. 1991;12(5):381–7.
22. Kamentsky LA, Gershman RJ, Kamentsky LD, Pomeroy BM, Weissman ML. CompuCyte Corporation. Pathfinder System: computerizing the microscope to improve cytology quality assurance. Acta Cytol. 1996;40(1):31–6.
23. Kamentsky LA, Burger DE, Gershman RJ, Kamentsky LD, Luther E. Slide-based laser scanning cytometry. Acta Cytol. 1997;41(1):123–43.
24. Kamentsky LA, Kamentsky LD, Fletcher JA, Kurose A, Sasaki K. Methods for automatic multiparameter analysis of fluorescence in situ hybridized specimens with a laser scanning cytometer. Cytometry. 1997;27(2):117–25.
25. Kamentsky LA. Laser scanning cytometry. Methods Cell Biol. 2001;63:51–87.
26. Tarnok A, Gerstner AO. Clinical applications of laser scanning cytometry. Cytometry. 2002;50(3):133–43.
27. Gerstner AO, Machlitt J, Welkoborsky HJ, Bootz F, Tarnok A. Analysis of ploidy in hypopharyngeal cancer by laser scanning cytometry on fine needle aspirate biopsies. Anal Cell Pathol. 2003;25(2):51–62.
28. Gerstner AO, Thiele A, Tarnok A, et al. Preoperative detection of laryngeal cancer in mucosal swabs by slide-based cytometry. Eur J Cancer. 2005;41(3):445–52.
29. Würflinger T, Stockhausen J, Meyer-Ebrecht D, Böcking A. Robust automatic coregistration, segmentation, and classification of cell nuclei in multimodal cytopathological microscopic images. Comput Med Imaging Graph. 2004;28(1–2):87–98.
30. Böcking A, Stockhausen J, Meyer-Ebrecht D. Towards a single cell cancer diagnosis. Multimodal and monocellular measurements of markers and morphology (5 M). Cell Oncol. 2006;26(1–2):73–9.
31. Remmerbach TW, Meyer-Ebrecht D, Aach T, et al. Toward a multimodal cell analysis of brush biopsies for the early detection of oral cancer. Cancer Cytopathol. 2009;117(3):228–35.
32. Rüschoff J, Plate K, Bittinger A, Thomas C. Nucleolar organizer regions (NORs). Basic concepts and practical application in tumor pathology. Pathol Res Pract. 1989;185(6):878–85.
33. Rüschoff J, Bittinger A, Neumann K, Schmitz-Moormann P. Prognostic significance of nucleolar organizing regions (NORs) in carcinomas of the sigmoid colon and rectum. Pathol Res Pract. 1990;186(1):85–91.

34. Rüschoff J. Nucleolus organizer regions in pathomorphologic tumor diagnosis. Veroff Pathol. 1992;139:1–144.
35. Aubele M, Biesterfeld S, Derenzini M, et al. Guidelines of AgNOR quantitation. Committee on AgNOR quantitation within the European Society of Pathology 1. Zentralbl Pathol. 1994;140(1):107–8.
36. Tuccari G, Giuffre G, Ofner D, Rüschoff J. Standardized use of the AgNOR method. J Oral Pathol Med. 2000;29(10):526–7.
37. Haroske G, Giroud F, Reith A, Böcking A. 1997 ESACP consensus report on diagnostic DNA image cytometry. Part I: basic considerations and recommendations for preparation, measurement and interpretation. European Society for Analytical Cellular Pathology. Anal Cell Pathol. 1998;17(4):189–200.
38. Würflinger T, Stockhausen J, Meyer-Ebrecht D, Böcking A. Automatic coregistration, segmentation and classification for multimodal cytopathology. Stud Health Technol Inform. 2003;95:218–23.
39. Bell A, Aach T, Ropers SO, Bocking A, Meyer-Ebrecht D, Wülflinger T. Towards fully automatic acquisition of multimodal cytopathological microscopy images with autofocus and scene managing. Methods Inf Med. 2007;46(3):314–23.
40. Rüschoff J. Nucleolus organizer regions in pathomorphologic tumor diagnosis. Veroff Pathol. 1992;139:1–144.
41. Crocker J, Boldy DA, Egan MJ. How should we count AgNORS? Proposals for a standardized approach. J Pathol. 1989;158(3):185–8.
42. Ploton D. Structure and molecular organization of the nucleolus. Zentralbl Pathol. 1994;140(1):3–6.
43. Ploton D, Bendayan M, Adnet JJ. Ultrastructural localization of Ag-NOR proteins and nucleic acids in reticulated nucleoli. Biol Cell. 1983;49(1):29–34.
44. Ploton D, Menager M, Jeannesson P, Himber G, Pigeon F, Adnet JJ. Improvement in the staining and in the visualization of the argyrophilic proteins of the nucleolar organizer region at the optical level. Histochem J. 1986;18(1):5–14.
45. Crocker J. Nucleolar organiser regions. Curr Top Pathol. 1990;82:91–149.
46. Remmerbach TW, Weidenbach H, Müller C, et al. Diagnostic value of nucleolar organizer regions (AgNORs) in brush biopsies of suspicious lesions of the oral cavity. Anal Cell Pathol. 2003;25(3):139–46.
47. Remmerbach TW, Hemprich A, Böcking A. Minimally invasive brush-biopsy: innovative method for early diagnosis of oral squamous cell carcinoma. Schweiz Monatsschr Zahnmed. 2007;117(9):926–40.
48. Maraki D, Becker J, Böcking A. Cytologic and DNA-cytometric very early diagnosis of oral cancer. J Oral Pathol Med. 2004;33(7):398–404.
49. Böcking A, Sproll C, Stocklein N, et al. Role of brush biopsy and DNA cytometry for prevention, diagnosis, therapy, and followup care of oral cancer. J Oncol. 2011;2011:875959.
50. Handschel J, Oz D, Pomjanski N, et al. Additional use of DNA-image cytometry improves the assessment of resection margins. J Oral Pathol Med. 2007;36(8):472–5.

Chapter 9
Diagnostic Cytometry

Alfred Böcking, David Friedrich, Chen Jin, André Bell, Thomas Würflinger, Dietrich Meyer-Ebrecht, Yu Zhang, Stefan Biesterfeld, Natalia Pomjanski, Leonid Berynskyy, Richard Yeung, Jörg Handschel, Branko Palcic, and Til Aach

Late Diagnosis of Oral Cancer

Patients with squamous cell carcinomas of the oral cavity currently have a fair prognosis with an overall 5-year survival rate of about 45% [1]. Unfortunately, this figure has not substantially improved during the past 30 years [2]. Late diagnosis resulting in late treatment and locoregional failure after surgery or even after combined surgery and irradiation are the main causes of death in patients with oral squamous cell carcinomas. Although mucosal biopsy is still regarded as the gold standard for definitive oral cancer diagnosis, exfoliative cytology is a valuable tool for the noninvasive evaluation of a range of potentially pre-neoplastic oral mucosa

Alfred Bocking and David Friedrich have contributed equally to this manuscript.

A. Böcking (✉)
Institute of Pathology, City-Hospital Düren, Roon Strasse 30, 52309 Düren, Germany
e-mail: boecking@uni-duesseldorf.de

D. Friedrich • A. Bell • T. Würflinger • D. Meyer-Ebrecht • Y. Zhang • T. Aach
Institute of Image Analysis and Computer Vision, RWTH Aachen University, Aachen, Germany

C. Jin • R. Yeung
Motic China Company, Xiamen, People's Republic of China

S. Biesterfeld • N. Pomjanski • L. Berynskyy
Institute of Cytopathology, Heinrich-Heine-University, Düsseldorf, Germany

J. Handschel
Department of Cranio- and Maxillofacial Surgery, Heinrich-Heine-University, Düsseldorf, Germany

B. Palcic
British Columbia Cancer Agency and University of British Columbia, Vancouver, Canada

R. Mehrotra (ed.), *Oral Cytology: A Concise Guide*, DOI 10.1007/978-1-4614-5221-8_9,

lesions, like leuko-/erythroplakias and lichen planus. As this noninvasive procedure is well tolerated by patients, more lesions may be screened and thus more oral cancers may be found in early, curable stages.

Early Diagnosis of Oral Cancer

Oral carcinogenesis proceeds through a stepwise accumulation of (cyto)genetic changes over time [1, 3]. Because the oral cavity is easy to examine and risk factors for oral cancer are known, there is a great opportunity/good chance to improve patient outcomes through early diagnosis and treatment of premalignant lesions before the development of invasive carcinomas [2, 4]. Oral premalignant lesions are morphologically abnormal solitary or multiple areas of mucosa that are typically white, red, speckled or verrucous in appearance. The WHO classification [2] combines leukoplakia and erythroplakia into 'precursor lesions', with a 6.8% estimated rate of transformation of oral leukoplakias to cancer. Oral lichen planus, a chronic inflammatory condition, also is associated with an increased risk of cancer development of about 3% [5, 6]. Early diagnosis within stages Tis or T1 corresponds to a vastly improved 5-year survival rate when compared with more advanced lesions (96.7%) [1, 2]. As this noninvasive procedure is well tolerated by patients, more lesions may be screened and thus more oral cancers may be found in early, curable stages.

Brush Biopsies in Screening

Screening for oral cancer and its precursor lesions may be performed by dentists, dental surgeons and other healthcare professionals. Exfoliative cytology, taking brush biopsies, is only advocated for evaluation of macroscopically suspicious lesions of the oral mucosa that are detected clinically by screening. Exfoliative cytology may replace tissue biopsy in lesions that are clinically not obviously suspicious for malignancy, but nevertheless need surveillance [4]. As tissue biopsy is associated with lower compliance by patients as compared to brush-biopsy, this non invasive approach may lead to a higher number of investigated suspicious oral lesions and thus to an increased rate of curable cancers, identified in their early stages.

Collection devices suitable to obtain cells from the superficial and intermediate layers of the oral mucosa may be conventional brushes, as used for endocervical sampling by gynecologists, such as the CytoBrush, Orca-brush or others. The brush is rotated under slight pressure several times on the suspicious lesion. Cells are then immediately smeared on glass slides and fixed with alcoholic spray. Morphological signs of dysplasia and malignancy will also be detected cytologically in the upper layers of the squamous epithelium due to the principle of migration of cells from basal to superficial layers. The degree of nuclear abnormality in the surface layers reflects the degree of disturbance of maturation of the whole thickness of the epithelium.

Assessment of Dysplasia

There are several schemes for grading dysplasia in biopsies of oral precursor lesions. The WHO classification provides a five step system: hyperplasia, mild, moderate and severe dysplasia followed by carcinoma in situ [6]. Squamous cell carcinoma may develop from antecedent dysplastic oral mucosal lesions—if an early diagnosis has not been made and treatment given. Early diagnosis within stages Tis or T1 corresponds to a vastly improved 5-year survival rate when compared with more advanced lesions (96.7%) [1, 4]. It is the task of cytopathologists to identify nuclear abnormalities in squamous cells to predict the histological grade of dysplasia. The diagnostic criteria used are well known and similar to those in cervical exfoliative cytology according to Papanicolaou [4]. Yet, the detection of dysplastic cells results in equivocal cytological diagnoses. Remmerbach et al. [1] reported a frequency of 13.9% doubtful or suspicious oral cytological diagnoses due to different grades of squamous dysplasia or abnormally regenerating epithelium. Although the degree of dysplasia can be predicted from cytological samples, tissue biopsy is usually performed when dysplasia is detected cytologically, to confirm its grade and exclude the presence of invasion. The latter cannot be reliably assessed by exfoliative cytology alone. However, poor interobserver reproducibility in the histological assessment of oral premalignant lesions is well described [8].

Accuracy of Oral Cytology

Cytopathologic evaluation of oral brush biopsies from leuko- and erythroplakias alone yields sensitivities for the detection of oral cancer slightly below those of histopathologic evaluation of scalpel biopsies, reported to be 97.5% [4]. Remmerbach et al. [1, 7] documented 91.3% resp. 94.6% sensitivity of oral brush biopsy and Maraki et al. [12] even 100% for the detection of oral cancer, including the in situ stage. Respective specificities were 99.5%, 95.1% resp. 97.4%. 28.6% of cancers were identified in early, curable stages Tis and T1 [1].

An accumulating body of evidence exists to show that oral cytology is a valuable technique for the assessment of oral premalignant lesions [1, 4–9]. Exfoliative cytology has been shown to detect dysplasia in suspicious oral lesions with high sensitivity and specificity by several groups [1, 4–9].

Up to 5–14% of oral brush biopsies may yield equivocal cytological diagnoses [1, 7]. Underlying diagnoses are mild, moderate or marked dysplasia, abnormal regenerating squamous epithelium or just scarcity of abnormal cells. In these cases, ancillary methods are desirable, that allow more definite, correct cytological diagnoses (see below).

Shortcomings of Oral Cytology

Exfoliative cytology has recently been shown to represent a valuable, noninvasive tool for the evaluation of oral leukoplakias, erythroplakias and lichen planus lesions [1, 4–11]. Yet, several problems currently preclude the propagation of conventional oral brush-biopsy as an adjuvant tool for screening to identify oral (pre)cancerous lesions:

(1) Diagnostic accuracy slightly below that of bioptic histology—might not be regarded as fully sufficient. (2) Interobserver reproducibility of cytologic assessment of oral squamous dysplasias will not be higher than that of their histological assessment. (3) In several countries, not enough cytodiagnostically skilled personnel are available to competently read an abundance of oral smears. In Germany e.g. most schools for cytotechnicians have been closed in the last decade. (4) The payment for time-consuming screening multiple smears per patient is insufficient in most countries, e.g. 8,- € currently in Germany. (5) The rate of 5–14% of equivocal cytological diagnoses results in too many scalpel biopsies for definitive assessment. (6) Identification of a few diagnostically relevant abnormal or atypical cells out of ten thousands of normal cells per slide is uneconomically time-consuming.

Meanwhile, auxiliary methods such as manual and automated DNA-image-cytometry (DNA-ICM) [1, 5, 7–9, 12], AgNOR-analysis [13, 14] and multimodal cell analysis [15] have been shown to increase diagnostic accuracy of oral cytology.

When and Why of DNA-Image Cytometry

DNA-ICM is based on microdensitometric DNA measurements in nuclei of several hundred atypical cells in routine cytological specimens. Cells are stained according to Feulgen, a stain where the uptake of stain in the nucleus is proportional to its DNA content. The DNA-content of nuclei can then be measured using a microscope with a digital camera, by measuring the attenuation of light on the whole nucleus area and calibrating the system on cells with normal DNA content, e.g. morphologically unsuspicious epithelial nuclei. In its conventional, *manual version* DNA-ICM aims at the identification of (prospectively) malignant cells out of microscopically atypical (dysplastic) or otherwise doubtful ones, in subjectively suspicious smears (Figs. 9.1, 9.3, 9.6). In its *automated version* it aims at screening an abundance of oral smears for the presence of atypical (dysplastic) or abnormal (malignant) cells and subsequent DNA-measurements on these only in order to identify definitely malignant ones (Figs. 9.2, 9.5, 9.8). The result of both modes of application is the exclusion or identification of DNA-aneuploidy as a specific marker for malignancy in squamous epithelial cells.

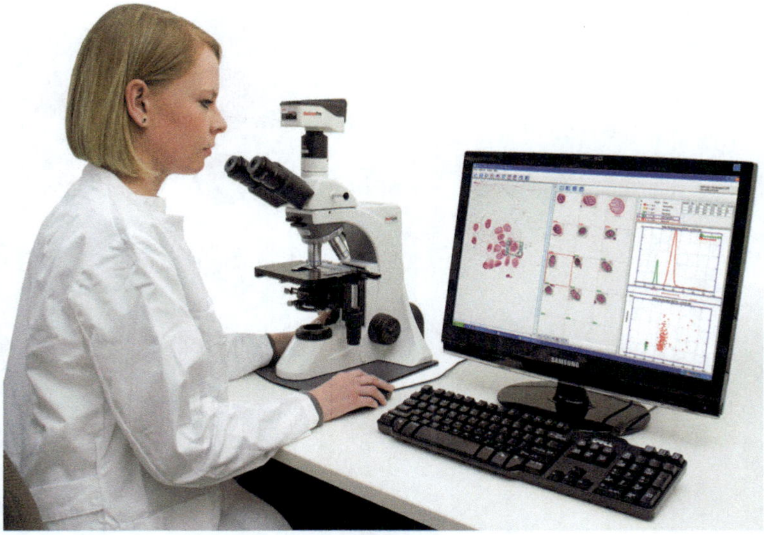

Fig. 9.1 MotiCyte-DNAi workstation with cytotechnician

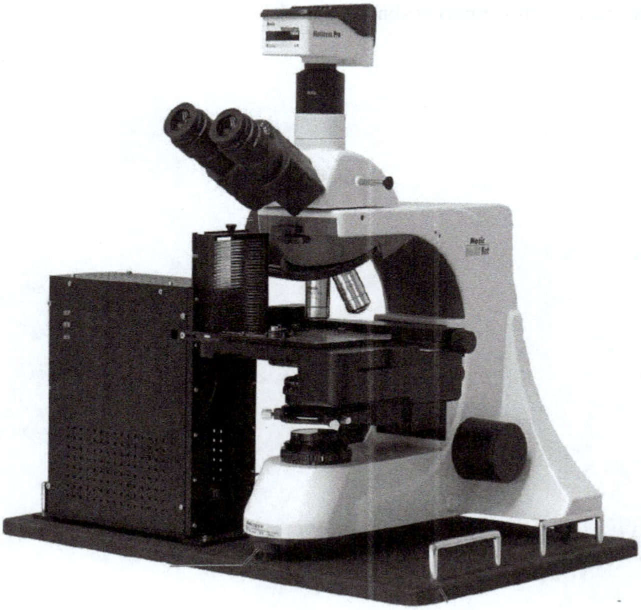

Fig. 9.2 MotiCyte-DNA-s screening system with slide loader

After enzymatic cell separation, DNA-ICM can also be applied on formalin-fixed and paraffin embedded tissues, i.e. on all histologic routine specimens like biopsies and resected tissues [11, 22]. Thus, even histologic diagnoses of dysplasias can be subjected to DNA-cytometry to predict their prospective behavior.

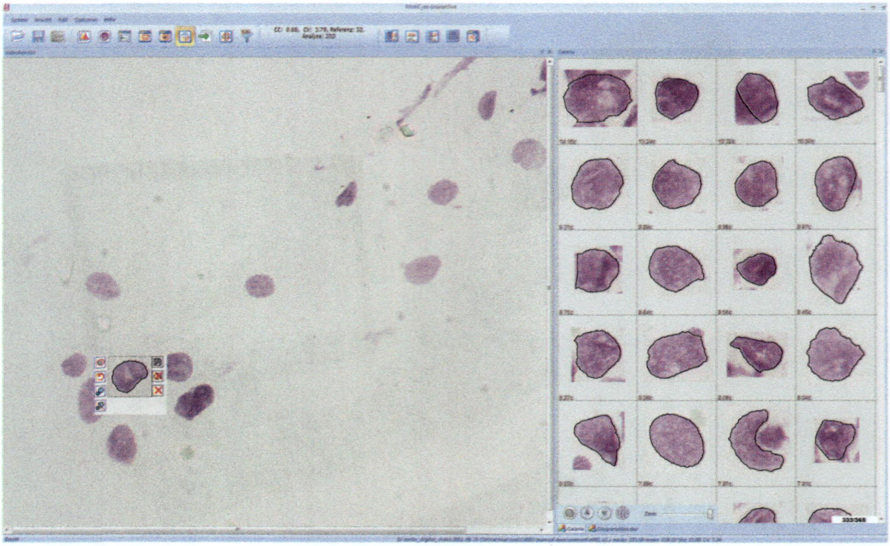

Fig. 9.3 Screen-shot MotiCyte-DNA-interactive, manual mode without classifier: Left: live image: Smear with five oral cancer cells one of them interactively selected and segmented (*black*). Right: Image gallery with segmented abnormal nuclei

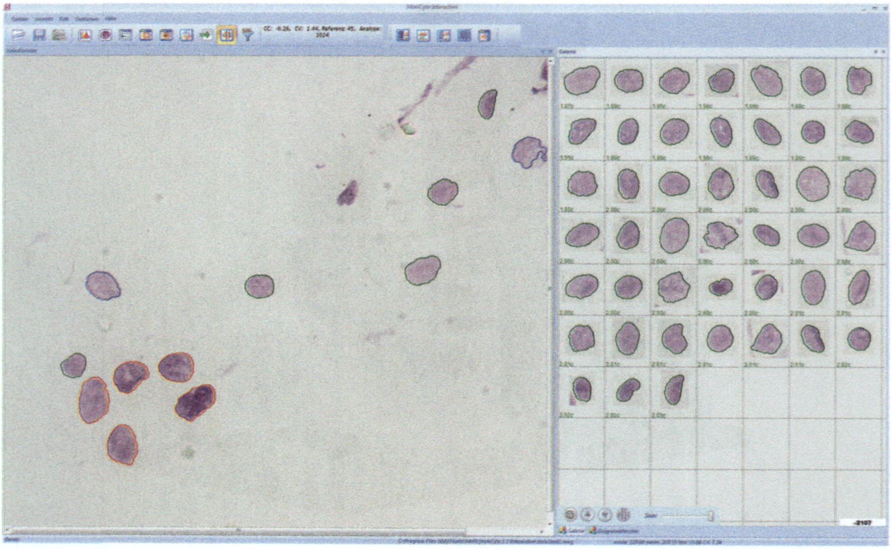

Fig. 9.4 Screen-shot MotiCyte-interactive, semi-automated mode with classifier: Left: life image: Smear with five cancer cells, automatically segmented and classified (*red*). Right: Image gallery with automatically classified normal epithelial cell nuclei

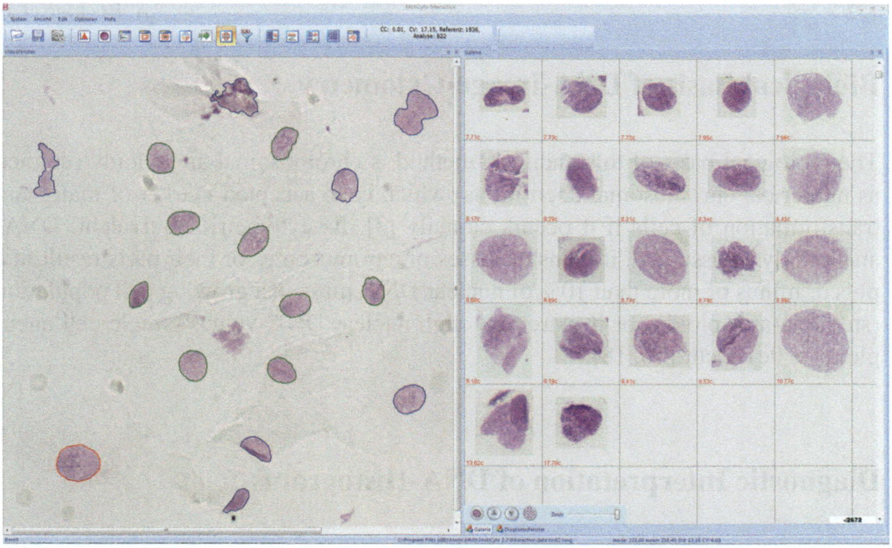

Fig. 9.5 Screen-shot MotiCyte-DNA-screener, automated classification mode: Left: live image: Smear with one oral cancer cell (*red*) and 15 normal nuclei, both automatically classified. Right: Image gallery with automatically classified abnormal nuclei

#		Count	Name	Min	Max	Mean	Mode	CV
0	A	440	abnormals	1.73	9.69	4.16	4.00	36.53
1	–	1035	Artefacts	0.16	9.77	2.43	0.00	79.63
2	–	9	Granulocytes	1.60	3.34	2.16	0.00	23.91
3	R	40	Norm. epithelial	1.98	2.01	2.00	2.00	0.42
4	–	1	Lymphocytes	2.10	2.10	2.10	0.00	0.00

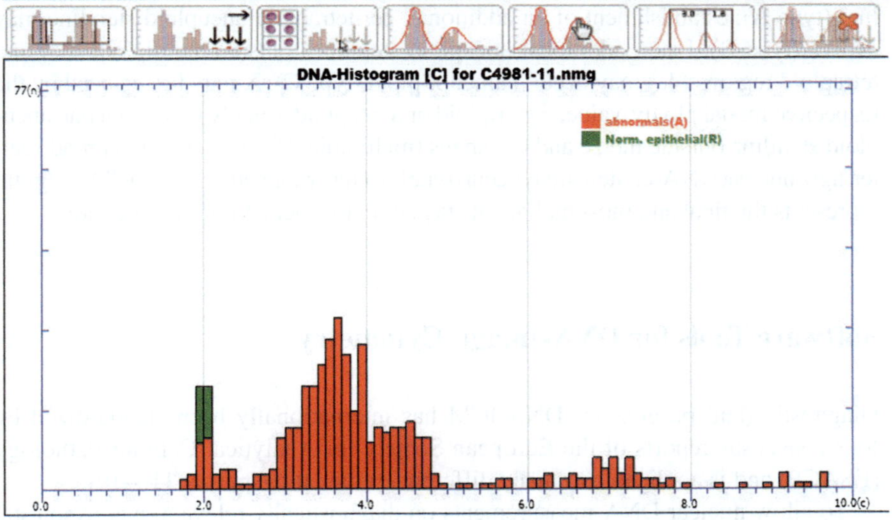

Fig. 9.6 Statistics (*above*) and multiploid-aneuploid DNA-histogram (*below*) from manual measurement (Fig. 9.3)

Biological Basis of DNA-Image-Cytometry

The biological basis of this ancillary method is chromosomal aneuploidy (defined as numerical chromosomal aberrations) which is an accepted marker of malignant transformation of cells if it occurs clonally [3]. Its cytometric equivalent, DNA-aneuploidy, is assumed, if gains or losses of chromosomes or their parts result in a plus or minus of more than 10% of nuclear DNA-mass in a growing cell population (stemline-aneuploidy) or if extremely high nuclear DNA-values (single-cell aneuploidy > 9c) occur [16, 18].

Diagnostic Interpretation of DNA-Histograms

Algorithms for identifying cancer cells by qualitative detection of DNA-aneuploidy differ from those that are used for grading malignancy by quantifying DNA-aneuploidy. DNA-stemline-aneuploidy is assumed if the modal values of stemlines lie outside of 2c, 4c or 8c ± 10% [16–18]. DNA-single-cell-aneuploidy is assumed, if single DNA-values are detected beyond a certain threshold. This depends on the occurrence and degree of euploid polyploidization in the respective tissue. As HPV-infection, irradiation and regeneration are capable to induce euploid tetraploidy and respective G2/M-phase cells may represent DNA-contents up to 8c, 9c is a reasonable threshold in oral mucosa to assume rare DNA-aneuploid cells, named 9c Exceeding Events, 9cEE [16–18]. The positive predictive value of stemline aneuploidy is higher than that of single-cell-aneuploidy alone [1, 5, 7–9].

As cytogenetic tumor progression proceeds, besides a peridiploid-aneuploid stemline (type A), establishment of an additional, peritetraploid-aneuploid stemline may evolve (type B). Later, additional aneuploid stemlines outside the diploid (2c) and tetraploid regions (4c) may occur, named x-ploid (type C). X may be replaced by the respective modal ploidy-value, e.g. triploid or heptaploid. Finally more than one aneuploid stemline outside the 2c and 4c ranges (multiploid, Fig. 9.6–9.8) and broad scattering of nuclear DNA-contents may occur (type D). This "Manhattan-Sykline"-histogram represents the final and most malignant stage of cytogenetic tumor progression.

Software Tools for DNA-Image-Cytometry

Diagnostic (and prognostic) DNA-ICM has internationally been standardized by four consensus reports of the European Society for Analytical Cellular Pathology (ESACP) and is applicable to many different epithelial dysplasias [16–19].

To allow nuclear DNA-measurements on diagnostically relevant, e.g. dysplastic or malignant cells, the final microscopic magnification and resolution should enable cytomorphologic assessment and differentiation of different types on the monitor

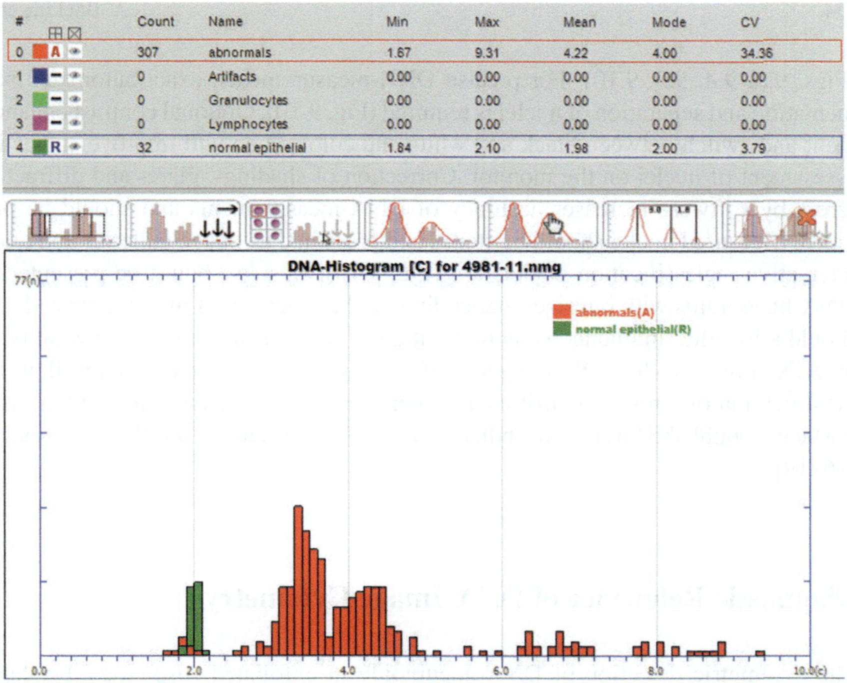

#		Count	Name	Min	Max	Mean	Mode	CV
0	A	307	abnormals	1.67	9.31	4.22	4.00	34.36
1	–	0	Artifacts	0.00	0.00	0.00	0.00	0.00
2	–	0	Granulocytes	0.00	0.00	0.00	0.00	0.00
3	–	0	Lymphocytes	0.00	0.00	0.00	0.00	0.00
4	R	32	normal epithelial	1.84	2.10	1.98	2.00	3.79

Fig. 9.7 Statistics (*above*) and similar multiploid-aneuploid DNA-histogram (*below*) from semiautomated measurement (Fig. 9.4)

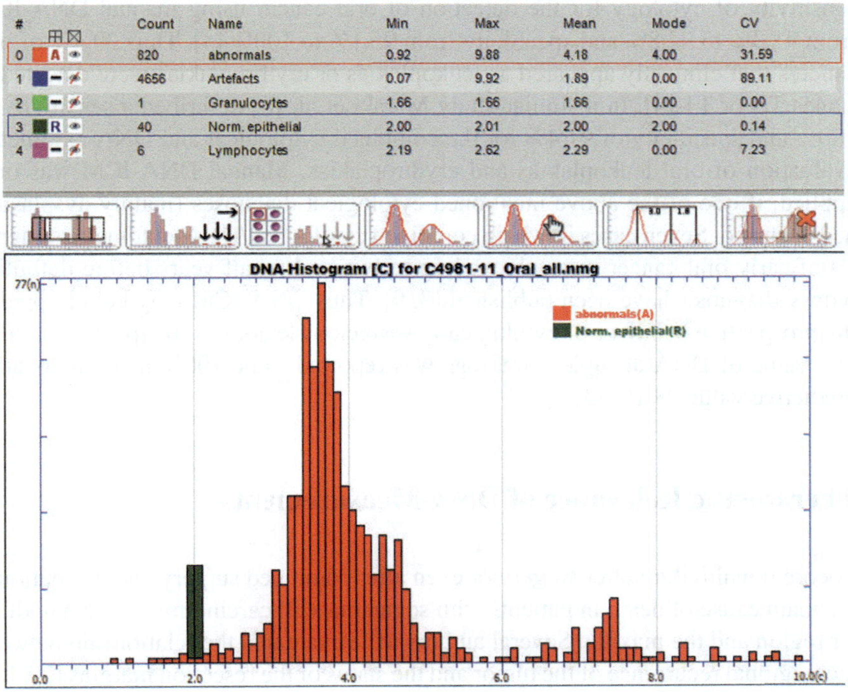

#		Count	Name	Min	Max	Mean	Mode	CV
0	A	820	abnormals	0.92	9.88	4.18	4.00	31.59
1	–	4656	Artefacts	0.07	9.92	1.89	0.00	89.11
2	–	1	Granulocytes	1.66	1.66	1.66	0.00	0.00
3	R	40	Norm. epithelial	2.00	2.01	2.00	2.00	0.14
4	–	6	Lymphocytes	2.19	2.62	2.29	0.00	7.23

Fig. 9.8 Statistics (*above*) and respective multiploid-aneuploid DNA-histogram (*below*) from automated measurement. (Fig. 9.5)

(Figs. 9.3, 9.4, 9.5, 9.10). For precise DNA-measurements, exact automated segmentation and separation of nuclei is required (Fig. 9.10). Optional contrast enhancement and switch between black and white and color-mode will improve subjective assessment of nuclei on the monitor. Correction of shading-, glare- and diffraction errors by software increases accuracy of DNA-measurements and should be provided. Measured nuclei should be stored and presented as image galleries and allow interactive reclassification or deletion (Fig. 9.10). Results should be presented as DNA-histograms with bin sizes, depending on the precision of measurement. These should allow the simultaneous representation of DNA-distribution for several types of cells (Figs. 9.6–9.8). Scatter plots of nuclear area vs. DNA-content allow the identification of errors of densitometric measurements. Diagnostically and/or prognostically published relevant indices of DNA-distribution should be provided [16–19].

Diagnostic Relevance of DNA-Image Cytometry

The cytometric detection of DNA-aneuploidy in exfoliated suspicious dysplastic oral cells qualifies these as malignant, up to 2 years earlier than cytology or histology alone [8, 9]. Applying DNA-aneuploidy as a marker for prospective malignancy on identical slides, Remmerbach and coworkers could improve diagnostic sensitivity of cytology for the detection of oral cancer using manual DNA-ICM from 91.3% to 97.8% and specificity from 95.1% to 100% [4]. Thus 29.4% of oral cancers that clinically appeared as leukoplakias or erythroplakias were detected in stages Tis or T1 [4]. In a similar study Maraki et al. [8] described a sensitivity of 100% and specificity of 97.4% for the combined cytological and DNA-cytometric evaluation of oral leukoplakias and erythroplakias. Manual DNA-ICM was only applied, if one of the above mentioned cytological diagnoses (mainly dysplasias) had occurred. Seven cases in which combined cytological/DNA-cytometric diagnosis of early oral cancer was achieved up to two and a half years before definitive biopsy diagnosis have been published [8, 9]. Thus DNA-ICM may help to predict the prospective behavior of cytologically suspicious lesions, as the positive predictive value of DNA-aneuploid findings was reported to be 100% and the negative predictive value 98.1% [4, 7].

Therapeutic Relevance of DNA-Measurements

Locoregional failure after surgery or even after combined surgery and irradiation is the main cause of death in patients with squamous cell carcinomas of the mandibular region and the maxilla. Several authors have evaluated the relationship between locoregional recurrence of the tumor and the status of the resection margins [20, 21]. The prevalence of tumoral infiltration at the resection margins is an indicator for additional excision, postoperative irradiation, and strict follow-up [20]. The recurrence rate in patients with positive margins of resection treated only by surgery ranges from 36% [21] to 64% [20]. Due to the fact that it can be difficult to distinguish between squamous cell carcinomas and other lesions of the oral mucosa, especially on frozen sections, the histological diagnosis of oral mucosa lesions sometimes fails [21]. The additional value of DNA-ICM regarding the early identification of locoregional remnants of cancer after resection was assessed by Handschel et al. [22]. In their study adjuvant use of DNA-ICM showed a high positive predictive value of 87.5% with respect to the prediction of local recurrence of head and neck squamous cell carcinomas. In conclusion, the additional use of DNA-image cytometry is a reasonable tool for the assessment of the resection margins of squamous cell carcinoma. DNA-ICM could help to find the appropriate treatment option for the patients and thus might improve their prognosis.

Automated DNA-Image-Cytometry

As we have seen, DNA Image Cytometry addresses shortcomings 1 (diagnostic accuracy slightly below histology) and 5 (unnecessary biopsies) mentioned above. Additionally, the diagnosis in DNA-ICM is not based on the subjective judgement of the morphology of nuclei, but on the measurement of nuclear DNA-contents, reducing interobserver variability (shortcoming 2). However, the fact that not enough skilled personnel are available (shortcoming 3), that reimbursements for this method do not cover expenses of the pathologists (shortcoming 4) or that screening for relevant cells is too time consuming (shortcoming 6), might cause that these benefits never to reach the patient.

One approach to reduce the workload for skilled personnel and to increase the objectivity of the method at the same time is to automate time consuming steps of the process of screening and measurement. Steps suitable for automation are the automated collection of nuclei in regions of interest as well as their pre-classification as belonging to different cell types. Therefore, the microscope is equipped with a motorized stage and objective revolver. After the regions of interest have been selected manually or detected by an algorithm, all nuclei in these regions are collected. During this collection, an autofocus procedure has to ensure that the nuclei are captured in focus. The collected nuclei are then pre-classified by a classification algorithm.

Nevertheless, during the whole process the diagnostic responsibility should remain in the hands of pathologists and full traceability of the process should be given. Therefore, it is required that a pathologist verifies the pre-classified digital nucleus classifications in diagnostically relevant cell groups and DNA ranges. Hence the workload of the pathologist is reduced to verifying these pre-classifications and finally performing the diagnosis on the DNA histogram and respective image galleries.

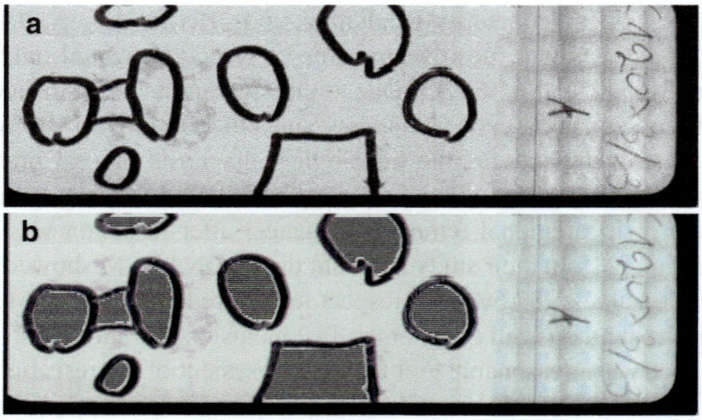

Fig. 9.9 (**a**) Stained oral smear with user-marked regions of interest, scanned under ×2 objective magnification and stitched together digitally. (**b**) Same maps scan as (**a**), where the areas of interest to be scanned marked were automatically detected and marked as hatched areas

Automated Selection of Regions of Interest

In most workflows of pathologies, applying diagnostic DNA-image-cytometry to brush smears of the oral mucosa, these are first examined in the conventional Papanicolaou-stain for identification of morphologically suspicious cells. These regions are marked with a felt tip pen on the glass slide. The slide is then restained according to Feulgen and felt tip markings are transferred back to the restained slide. DNA-ICM measurements are finally performed within these regions only. To emulate this workflow also for the automated scan, algorithms for the automated detection of those regions which are encircled by felt tip markers are required.

For this purpose, an overview is created by scanning the slide under 2× objective-magnification, digitally stitching together the images and converting them into a gray level image (Fig. 9.9a). The interior of the felt tip marker regions is then detected by the following procedure:

1. Identification of slide-label position by deciding whether the left or the right side of the image is darker.
2. Identification of marker-lines by an adaptive thresholding algorithm on the image, excluding the slide label area.
3. Filtering out detected regions which are too small to belong to a felt tip marker region.
4. Filling of the interior areas of the detected felt-tip marker lines.
5. Subtracting image of step 3 from image of step 4.
6. Transferring the regions found to the original image (Fig. 9.9b).

Due to the gray level conversion of the image and the adaptive thresholding algorithm used for detecting the felt tip marker lines, this procedure can deal with a variety of marker colors such as red, blue, green and black—they all yield dark regions in the gray level image. As the slide label is detected automatically, the user can put the label on either side and the system reacts to this. The proposed procedure saves the time for manually selecting the regions of interest. Even more importantly, in combination with an automated slide loader, this algorithm enables the successive scan of dozens of slides in a row without manual interaction. The system can then run overnight as well, which improves its economic use (shortcoming 4).

Autofocus Strategies

Next the system switches to a higher magnification which is needed for screening the cells in the selected regions of interest, e.g. with a 40× objective. The microscope steers to all relevant areas in the regions of interest and automatically collects all the nuclei.

An important part of the automated cell collection is the autofocus procedure. Since the depth of field of the microscope is low, especially at high magnifications, the position of best focus might even change for scenes in close proximity. However, overlooking cancerous cells because they are out of focus must be prevented. Therefore, methods for automatically and robustly ensuring that the scenes are always in focus are necessary.

Autofocus Score

As a basis, a focus score for each region under examination is required, which assigns higher scores to area in focus than to defocused ones. As in well focused images, the objects often show clear boundaries which are smoother in defocused images, edge detection algorithms can be used for focus assessment. The edge detection methods of Roberts and Sobel as well as a Laplacian based method have been implemented in MotiCyte [23].

In the MotiCyte Screener system (Fig. 9.2), two autofocus functions are available: Field Focus Level Search and Interpolated Focus Map.

The Field Focus Level Search performs an autofocus on each field of view during scanning. The procedure is based on the focus position of the previously scanned field of view. The focus scores of images taken from neighboring z values, both with higher and lower z value, are computed and form a focus curve. This curve has a maximum peak and the z position belonging to this maximum is chosen as best focus position. Usually three to six movements for the field focus position search are used for finding the best focus position. In an alternative scanning mode, the Interpolated Focus Map, the position of best focus is estimated from a few positions in focus, which saves the time for focusing separately on each field of view. To this end, a certain number of focus points is defined from previously detected cell regions, evenly distributed over the slide. Subsequently, a focus procedure is performed on these defined points to obtain the best focus position for each of these points. Based on the *x*, *y* and *z* position of these focus points, a Delaunay triangulation algorithm is used to generate a group of fixed and flattened triangulations which cover the whole cell area and interpolate the 3D surface of the slide. The focus level of any field of view in the scanning area can then be computed as follows: Based on the *x*/*y* coordinate of field to be scanned, the triangulation to which the field belongs is found and the *z* level is calculated based on the plane which can be fitted through the three corner points of the triangle. The system moves to this estimated *z* position and all nuclei in the field of view are collected. The number of focus points N can be selected based on the smoothness of the slide surface and generally ranges from 6 to 20 points.

By using one of these two methods, there is no need for autofocus hardware and a sufficiently good focus quality can be achieved.

Scanning Speed

The color-camera pixel resolution in MotiCyte-systems is 1,360 × 1,024 and each pixel measures 0.18 microns at 40× resolution. Therefore each image covers an area of 245 × 184 microns so that scanning a 10 × 10 mm slide area, covered by cells is equivalent to capture 2,200 images. MotiCyte-DNA-screener can automatically scan the slide, including stage-movement, autofocus, nuclear segmentation and classification at 5 frames per second. Thus the process of capturing and processing 2,200 fields takes about 7 min.

Automated Pre-classification

Feulgen stained slides from oral brush smears usually contain, apart from artifacts, nuclei of granulocytes, lymphocytes and epithelial cells. The latter can be divided further into normal, atypical with suspicious (dysplastic) and abnormal (cancer) epithelial cells with unequivocally malignant nuclear morphology. In order to automate DNA Image Cytometry, the task of differentiating these nuclei has to be taught to a computer. The gap to be closed is the "language difference" between pathologists and the computer. While a pathologist would, for instance, describe the nucleus of a granulocyte as an object which is rather small, dark and has a segmented shape, the machine itself works with logical and mathematical operations and strictly follows the programmed algorithms. In order to "translate" the decision or classification process of the pathologist, the following three components were used:

1. A total of 35,920 objects were collected from ten oral smears and classified by a pathological expert (A. B.) into the five cellular classes of types, mentioned above. This so called gold standard is used as a database, so that the machine can look up how the pathologist classified objects from representative clinical smears. The objects originated from two tumor cell-negative specimens, one suspicious for malignancy (containing mild and moderately

dyskaryotic nuclei) with subsequent euploid DNA distribution, three suspicious with subseq uent DNA-aneuploidy, and four tumor cell-positive smears.

2. A set of 18 feature descriptors for Feulgen stained nuclei was implemented [24, 25]. The aim of these descriptors is to find numerical values representing diagnostic criteria which are used by cytopathologists to classify nuclei from different cell types and probabilities to represent cancer cells. These features finally quantify conventional empiric nuclear diagnostic features, such as size, shape, chromasia and chromatin-pattern.
3. A classifier was trained based on the gold standard database and the feature descriptors. Generally speaking, for an unknown object to be classified, the feature descriptors from two are computed and then the most likely class for such feature values, as learned from the gold standard, is assigned. In this example, a combination of decision trees is used for that purpose.

Classification Performance

To evaluate the performance of the classifier, a so called Leaving-one-out strategy was used. For objects from ten different slides, the diagnostic classifications are known. Objects from nine slides are considered as known to the computer. The objects from the remaining slide are then classified using the nine slides as the Gold standard reference database. The classification outcome is then compared to the pathologist's classification. This procedure is repeated such that each slide is classified once, correct and misclassifications are then summed for the final result. It can be shown that this process gives a close estimate of the classification performance of the final classifier, which uses all ten slides as reference database [26].

The classification performance is displayed in Table 9.1. The classifier achieves a total correct nuclear classification rate of 91.52%. Yet, the diagnosis in DNA Image Cytometry finally is based on the DNA content of hundreds of morphologically atypical and abnormal epithelial cell nuclei. Therefore, misclassifications which are especially relevant for diagnosis are:

- The misclassification of nuclei which are, in truth, abnormal (missed atypical and abnormals): If these abnormal cells are not included, this might lead to a false negative diagnosis. The rate of abnormals/atypicals lost among all abnormal/atypical nuclei is 7.14% on average (see Table 9.1).
- The classification of artifacts as abnormal/atypical nuclei. While granulocytes, lymphocytes and normal epithelial cells have normal DNA content and cannot lead to the diagnosis of cancer if misclassified as abnormal/atypical, artifacts such as dirt or overlapping nuclei are often assigned critical DNA-values. Therefore, artifacts classified as abnormals might lead to a false positive diagnosis. The rate of artifacts classified as abnormals/atypicals among all nuclei which the classifier classified as abnormal is 4.5% (see Table 9.1).

Table 9.1 Classification by pathological expert

		Abnormals	Artifacts	Granulocytes	Lymphocytes	Normal epithel
Automated classification	Abnormals	4,174	176	0	1	23
	Artifacts	268	20,877	969	187	321
	Granulocytes	3	694	3,379	34	1
	Lymphocytes	5	65	23	537	24
	Norm. epithel	45	163	12	30	3,909
	Total	4,495	21,975	4,383	789	4,278
	Error (in %)	7.14	5.00	22.91	31.94	8.63

Safety Net

As the aim of the presented system is to reduce the workload for cytotechnicians and cytopathologists, but never to remove the responsibility for diagnosis from the pathologist, a safety net procedure is advisable in the workflow for automated diagnostic DNA-Image Cytometry: After nuclei have been automatically collected and pre-classified, the pathologist is asked to check all abnormal/atypical nuclei and all artifacts in the diagnostically relevant ranges (exceeding events and abnormal stemlines). For this safety net procedure, the nuclei are presented in a gallery (Fig. 9.7) and the pathologist may delete or reclassify misclassified nuclei.

Diagnostic Performance

To evaluate the performance of automated diagnostic DNA-Image-Cytometry, nuclei from ten slides were automatically collected, pre-classified and the safety net procedure described above was applied. The slides included smears from two negative, four tumor cell-positive and four suspicious specimens. From the suspicious specimens, two were DNA-euploid and two DNA-aneuploid in a manual DNA-ICM measurement. The diagnoses concerning presence or absence of DNA-aneuploidy as defined earlier in the passages on "Diagnostic and prognostic interpretation of DNA-histograms" could be confirmed in all ten cases. The number of abnormal/atypical nuclei which needed to be interactively verified was seven on average, the number of artifacts to be verified was 110 per case.

Applying the described methods for automated nucleus collection and pre-classification, three different workflows become available:

- Conventional manual DNA-ICM: Manual scene selection and manual cell classification (Figs. 9.1, 9.3 and 9.6)
- Semi-Interactive DNA-ICM: Manual scene selection and automated cell collection (Figs. 9.1, 9.4 and 9.7)
- Automated DNA-ICM: Automated scene selection and automated cell collection (Figs. 9.2, 9.5, 9.8).

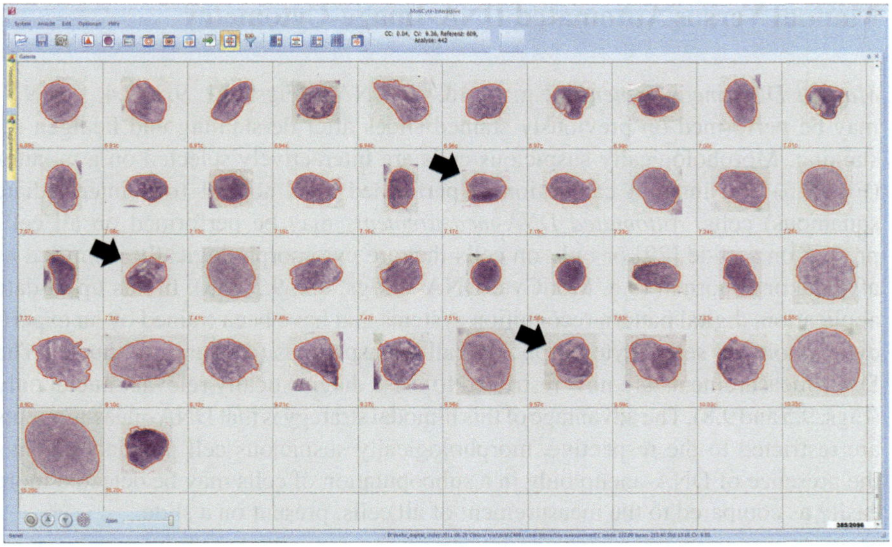

Fig. 9.10 Screen-shot after automated classification representing abnormal nuclei with five errors (artifacts) to be manually deleted

Pre-classification of nuclei is performed by a combination of decision trees and achieved a correct classification rate of 91.52% as compared to the expert (A.B.). This classification rate plus the safety net procedure was sufficient to obtain nearly identical DNA-histograms (Figs. 9.6–9.8) that resulted in identical final diagnoses in all ten cases relating to the presence or absence of DNA-aneuploid cancer cells. The automation processes described can actually be compared to the work of a harvester-thresher in agriculture: Similar to the harvester-thresher, which cuts the crops and separates the wheat from the chaff, these methods automatically collect nuclei and select the morphologically relevant ones for DNA-cytometry-based diagnosis. As the objects/nuclei which need to be checked after collection are compactly presented in an image gallery (Fig. 9.10), the interaction time is reduced from approximately 40 min to 10 min per measurement.

Another essential component of this approach is that our nuclear classifier is able to distinguish between morphologically normal and atypical and abnormal (dysplastic & malignant) epithelial nuclei. This means that the machine solves the "needle in the haystack"-problem, that is to find a minority of atypical/abnormal cell nuclei (e.g. 400/slide) in a majority of those from normal epithelial and inflammatory cells (e.g. 50,000/slide). If all epithelial nuclei were used for diagnosis, the atypical and abnormal nuclei might "drown in the mass" of the normal nuclei. But with this classification available, the diagnosis can now be based on the DNA content of abnormal and atypical nuclei only, which increases diagnostic performance of the method. Furthermore, the time needed for the measurement is significantly reduced.

Manual Versus Automated DNA-Image-Cytometry

Manual DNA-measurements (e.g. MotiCyte-DNA-i, Figs. 9.1, 9.3, 9.4, 9.6, 9.7) may be performed on previously stained slides after de-staining and Feulgen re-staining. Morphologically suspicious cells are interactively selected on a monitor (Fig. 9.3) and internal calibration is performed with normal (e.g. intermediate squamous) cells. *Automated DNA-measurements* may be performed on all cells present on a slide [29] or only on cells that are cytomorphologically identified as atypical or abnormal (e.g. MotiCyte-DNA-s, Figs. 9.2, 9.5, 9.8). In this up-to-date application, digital pattern recognition systems that have been trained by an expert-cytopathologist select cytomorphologically conspicuous (dyskaryotic) nuclei. The DNA-measurements are now restricted to these diagnostically relevant nuclei only (Figs. 9.5 and 9.8). The advantage of this bimodal strategy is that DNA-measurements are restricted to the respective, morphologically suspicious cell population. Thus the presence of DNA-aneuploidy in a subpopulation of cells may be detected more easily as compared to the measurement of all cells, present on a slide.

Approval for DNA-Cytometry-Devices

Devices for nuclear DNA-measurements that will be used for diagnostic and/or prognostic interpretations of human specimens should fulfill respective international medical performance standards, as those of the European Society for Analytical Cellular Pathology (ESACP, 16–19). Furthermore, approvals as in-vitro-diagnostic medical devices, issued by national or international authorities, as the US Food and Drug Administration (FDA) or the European Community (EC-label) should be documented for commercially available devices.

AgNOR-Analysis

Another auxiliary method that allows assessment of potential malignancy of dysplastic or regenerating cells is AgNOR-analysis. AgNORs represent silver-stainable nucleolar organizer regions. Their number and size is related to protein synthesis. Remmerbach et al. [10, 12] showed that counting the number of silver nitrate stained nucleolar organizer regions (AgNORs) in about 100 atypical squamous cells allows 100% sensitivity and specificity of oral cancer detection on brush biopsies. Both methods, DNA-ICM and AgNOR-analysis, may even be performed sequentially on identical cells. This type of multimodal cell analysis is especially useful, if only few atypical cells are available [12]. Thus, AgNOR-analysis can be combined with DNA-ICM if the latter does not yield an unequivocal diagnosis.

Current Automated Diagnostic Devices

The USA-device Oral CDx, using neuronal-network technology, aims at the identification of morphologically suspicious cells in conventionally stained brush-biopsy smears that require subsequent bioptic assessment [27, 28]. The Canadian Cyto-Savant system [29] automatically measures DNA-contents and chromatin texture features in Feulgen-stained nuclei of all epithelial cells per slide. The Chinese-German MotiCyte-DNA-interactive system allows DNA-measurements on manually selected or on digitally classified cells. MotiCyte-DNA-s automatically screens whole slides and measures DNA selectively on digitally pre-classified abnormal and atypical cells only. Both the Canadian and Chinese-German systems aim at definite diagnoses, based on the presence (cancer cells) and absence (no cancer cells) of DNA-aneuploidy per smear [29].

Summary

While oral lesions, that macroscopically are highly suspicious for cancer, should be submitted to scalpel-biopsy and histologic evaluation, the majority of facultatively precancerous lesions, such as leuko- and erythroplakias or even persistent lichen planus lesions, may be assessed by brush-biopsy and cytology. As this non-invasive procedure is well tolerated by patients, more lesions may be screened and thus more oral cancers may be found in early, curable stages. Oral brush-biopsies can easily be performed by dentists, dental surgeons and general practitioners. While sensitivity of exfoliative cytology alone is about 4% lower than bioptic histology, the combination of the latter with DNA-image-cytometry reaches the same diagnostic accuracy as the former (sensitivity 97.8–100%, specificity, 97.4–100%). As clonal chromosomal- and DNA-aneuploidy mostly precede cytological and histological evidence of malignancy in the squamous epithelium, its detection allows the diagnosis of oral squamous cell carcinomas up to 2 years earlier. Moreover, the additional use of DNA-image cytometry is a reasonable tool for the assessment of the resection margins of squamous cell carcinomas. DNA-image-cytometry could help to find the appropriate treatment option for patients and thus might improve their prognosis. Diagnostic DNA-image-cytometry is an objective method and has internationally been standardized.

Here, for the first time, we describe the performance of a device for automated screening of oral brush-biopsy-smears, based on a cascaded diagnostic strategy: (1) Automated selection of morphologically suspicious nuclei, (2) Interactive control and correction of these on digital image galleries, (3) DNA-measurements on these, (4) Final diagnosis on DNA-histograms and nuclear morphology.

References

1. Remmerbach W, Mathes SN, Weidenbach H, et al. Non invasive brush biopsy as an innovative tool for early detection of oral carcinomas. Mund Kiefer Gesichtschir. 2004;8(4):229–36.
2. Sciubba JJ. Oral cancer. The importance of early diagnosis and treatment. Am J Clin Dermatol. 2001;2(4):239–51.
3. Duesberg P, Mandrioli D, McCormack A, Nicholson M. Is carcinogenesis a form of speciation? Cell Cycle. 2011;10(13):2100–14.
4. Mehrotra R, Gupta DK. Exciting new advances in oral cancer diagnosis: avenues to early detection. Head Neck Oncol. 2011;10(13):2100–14.
5. Maraki D, Yalcinkaya S, Pomjanski N, et al. Cytologic and DNA-cytometric examination of oral lesions in lichen planus. J Oral Pathol Med. 2006;35(4):227–32.
6. Mehrotra R, Hullamnn M, Smeets R, Reichert TE, et al. Oral cytology revisited. J Oral Pathol Med. 2009;38(2):161–6.
7. Remmerbach TW, Weidenbach H, Hemprich A, et al. Cytologic and DNA-cytometric early diagnosis of oral cancer. Anal Cell Pathol. 2001;22(4):211–21.
8. Maraki D, Becker J, Böcking A. Cytologic and DNA-cytometric very early diagnosis of oral cancer. J Oral Pathol Med. 2004;33(7):398–404.
9. Remmerbach TW, Weidenbach H, Müller C, et al. Earliest detection of oral cancer using non-invasive brush biopsy including DNA-image-cytometry: report on four cases. Anal Cell Pathol. 2003;25(4):159–66.
10. Sloan P, Böcking A. Oral cavity. In: Gray W, Kocjan G, editors. Gray's diagnostic cytopathology. Churchill Livingstone, 3rd. ed., Edinburgh; 2010. p 297–308.
11. Böcking A, Sproll C, Naujoks C, et al. Role of brush biopsy and DNA-cytometry for prevention, diagnosis, therapy and followup care of oral cancer. J Oncol. 2011:Article ID 875959.
12. Klanrit P, Sperandio M, Brown AL, et al. DNA ploidy in proliferative verrucous leukoplakia. Oral Oncol. 2007;43(3):310–6.
13. Remmerbach TW, Weidenbach H, Müller C, et al. Diagnostic value of nucleolar organizer regions (AgNORs) in brush biopsies of suspicious lesions of the oral cavity. Anal Cell Pathol. 2003;25(3):139–46.
14. Bell A, Brauers J, Kaftan JN, et al. High dynamic range microscopy for cytopathological cancer diagnosis. IEEE J Sel Top Sig Proc. 2009;3(1):170–84 (Special issue on: digital image processing techniques for oncology).
15. Remmerbach TW, Meyer-Ebrecht D, Aach T, et al. Toward a multimodal cell analysis of brush biopsies for the early detection of oral cancer. Cancer Cytopathol. 2009;117(3):228–35.
16. Böcking A, Giroud F, Reith A. Consensus report of the ESACP task force on standardization of diagnostic DNA image cytometry. European Society for Analytical Cellular Pathology. Anal Cell Pathol. 1995;8(1):67–74.
17. Haroske G, Baak JPA, Danielesen H, et al. Fourth updated ESACP consensus report on diagnostic DNA image cytometry. Anal Cell Pathol. 2001;23(2):89–95.
18. Haroske G, Giroud F, Reith A, et al. 1997 ESACP consensus report on diagnostic DNA-image-cytometry. Part I: basic considerations and reccommendations for preparation, measurement and interpretation. Anal Cell Pathol. 1998;17:189–200.
19. Giroud F, Haroske G, Reith A, et al. 1997 ESACP consensus report on diagnostic DNA-image-cytometry. Part II: specific reccommendations for quality assurance. Anal Cell Pathol. 1998;17:201–8.
20. Ravasz LA, Slootweg JP, Hordijk GJ, et al. The status of the resection margin as a prognostic factor in the treatment of head and neck carcinoma. J Craniomaxillofac Surg. 1991;19(7):314–8.
21. Spiro RH, Guillamondegui O, Paulno AF, et al. Pattern of invasion and margin assessment in patients with oral tongue cancer. Head Neck. 1999;21(5):408–13.
22. Handschel J, Öz D, Pomjanski N, et al. Additional use of DNA-image cytometry improves the assessment of resection margins. J Oral Pathol Med. 2007;36(8):472–530.
23. Gonzalez RC, Woods RE. Digital image processing. Prentics Hall International. 3rd ed. 2008.

24. Rodenacker K, Bengtson E. A feature set for cytometry on digitized microscopic images. Anal Cell Pathol. 2003;25:1–36.
25. Holmquist E, Bengtson O, Eriksson O. Computer analysis of cervical cells: automatic feature extraction and classification. J Histochem Cytochem. 1978;26:1000–17.
26. Fukunaga K. Introduction to statistical pattern recognition. 2nd ed. Academic Press, Inc., San Diego, CA; 1990, p. 26.
27. Neher A, Öfner G, Appenroth E, et al. High resolution image cytometry on smears of normal oral mucosa: a possible approach for the early detection of laryngopharyngeal cancers. Head Neck. 2004;26(8):694–700.
28. Scheifele C, Schmidt-Westhausen AM, Dietrich T, et al. The sensitivity and specificity of the OralCDx technique: evaluation of 103 cases. Oral Oncol. 2004;40:824–8.
29. Garner DM, et al. The CytoSavant™ and its use in automated screening of cervical smears. In: Wied GL et al., editors. Compendium on the compuetrized cytology and histology laboratory. Chicago, Illinois: Tutorials of Cytology; 1994. p. 346–52.

Chapter 10
Pitfalls and Limitations of Oral Cytopathology

Anshul Singh, Deborah J. Carroll, and Ravi Mehrotra

A useful diagnostic technique should be easy to use, cause minimal discomfort, and have the capacity to collect sufficient material for analysis [1]. Ideally, a diagnostic procedure should be neither time-consuming nor complicated and in addition to high sensitivity, should also have high specificity. Cytology optimally meets all of these requirements, particularly when it is supplemented by an adequate image-analysis method [2]. However, the cytopathologist reading the smears and the clinician interpreting the results should be aware of certain pitfalls and gray zones inherent to the technique. This chapter endeavors to provide a brief review of some of these issues.

Exfoliative cytology for screening of oral cancer and pre-cancer has never achieved the same success as it has in cervical screening. This method proved to have low sensitivity in the diagnosis of oral cancer [3–5]. Exfoliative cytology performed on oral cancers has high false negative rates, which can exceed 30%. Furthermore, the effectiveness of exfoliative cytology for detecting dysplasia has false negative rates as high as 63% [6]. The reported high rate of false negatives was attributed to several factors including inadequate sampling, a high risk of procedural errors, and the subjective interpretation of the findings [7].

The adaptation of the cytobrush for oral cancer diagnoses helped revive major interest in oral cytology. Since then, various studies have been published describing different diagnostic techniques that have improved the sensitivity and specificity of conventional oral cytology [8, 9]. The main pitfalls and limitations are:

A. Singh (✉)
Department of Pathology, Moti Lal Nehru Medical College,
176/C/59C, Tagore town, Allahabad, Uttar Pradesh 211002, India
e-mail: anshul.sjh@gmail.com

D.J. Carroll
Oral CDx Laboratories, 2 Executive Boulevard, Suite 102, Suffern, NY 10901, USA

R. Mehrotra
Institute of Cytology and Preventive Oncology (ICPO), I-7, Sector - 39, Noida - 201301, Uttar Pradesh, India
e-mail: rm8509@gmail.com

R. Mehrotra (ed.), *Oral Cytology: A Concise Guide*, DOI 10.1007/978-1-4614-5221-8_10,

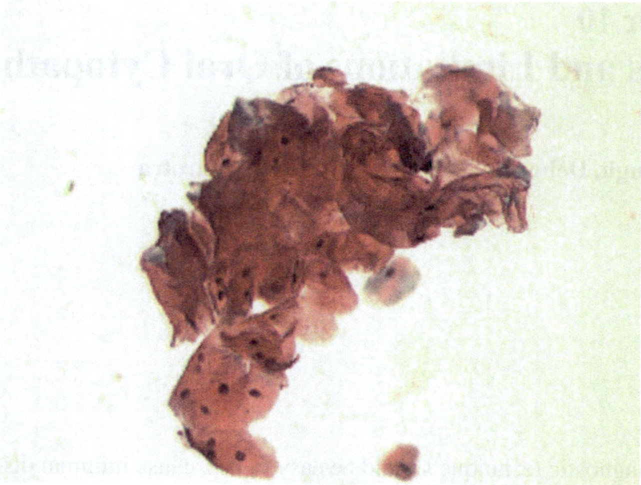

Fig. 10.1 Keratotic lesions: The sample consisted of only anucleate keratinocytes and superficial cells as shown. The histopathology of the lesion showed well differentiated squamous cell carcinoma

1. *Selection of site*—Dysplasia and early curable oral cancers are lesions that may easily be overlooked and neglected [10]. Most of them have a deceptively innocuous appearance and may not induce sufficient clinical concern to prompt further investigation. This failure to sample may result in the unfortunate loss of an opportunity to identify and treat potentially curable lesions at an early stage.
2. *Inaccessible sites*—Lesions in areas such as the posterior oropharynx and tonsils which are not easily accessible may be missed altogether.
3. *Lesion characteristics*—Certain changes associated with the lesion can lead to inadequate sampling. These include:

   (a) *Keratosis*—A thick hyperkeratotic layer may hinder sampling of lesions by prohibiting access to the deeper tissues where the malignant changes are most likely to be present, leading to failure in diagnosis. Unless the keratosis is associated with an ulcerated or erythematous area or an effort is made to remove surface anucleate cells prior to sampling, the value of cytology is limited. Specimens will usually consist predominantly or exclusively of anucleate keratinocytes and anucleate plaques, or sampling may yield only paucicellular smears (Fig. 10.1).

   (b) *Ulcerated lesions*—There is a tendency to sample the center of ulcers because of the relative ease of obtaining material from this area. This should be avoided because such samples consist predominantly of fibrinopurulent exudate, blood, and necrotic material which may obscure the rare diagnostic cells. Care should be taken to sample the margins (Fig. 10.2).

   (c) *Infections*—Abnormal cells may be difficult to detect in the midst of numerous cells exhibiting reactive or reparative changes which may be seen in infection with inflammation of the superficial layers.

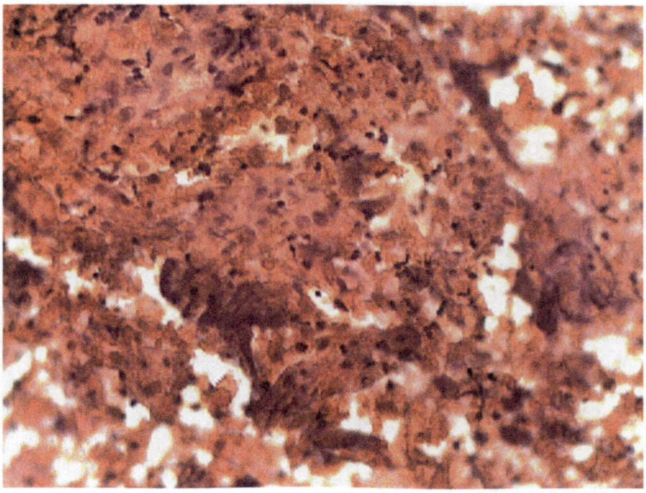

Fig. 10.2 Ulcerated lesions: the smear of the lesion showed inflammatory cells, blood and fibrinopurulent exudate with superficial cells, and was insufficient for analysis

4. *Procedural errors*:

   (a) *Superficial sampling*—This may be the result of either unfavorable lesion characteristics as described above or poor sampling technique, such as performing too few passes with the brush over the lesion.
   (b) Inadequate transfer of all the cells onto the glass slide will reduce the amount of material available for analysis, and consequently decrease the likelihood that the relevant pathology will be identified.
   (c) Obscuring of cellular material by non-cellular elements such as debris, food, mucus, and/or bacteria which were not removed prior to obtaining the smear (Fig. 10.3).
   (d) Improper smear technique resulting in either excessive smear thickness with excessive overlap of cells or smearing artifact, resulting in cellular distortion (Figs. 10.4 and 10.5).
   (e) Air drying artifact—may significantly impact evaluation of nuclear and cytoplasmic features and is a major problem for interpretation of cytology specimens from any location (Fig. 10.6).
   (f) Poor staining of the smear—may occur due to failure of the Pap stain as a result of improper water pH, exhaustion of stains, expired reagents, inadvertent exposure of the slide to formalin, or overheating of the slide during drying. In such cases, important diagnostic information regarding cytoplasmic differentiation and nuclear details may be lost (Fig. 10.7).

4. *Interpretation errors*—Expertise and relevant experience in the interpretation of oral cytopathology is a requirement that can not be overemphasized. Diagnostic errors on the part of the cytopathologist can lead to false negatives as well as false positives.

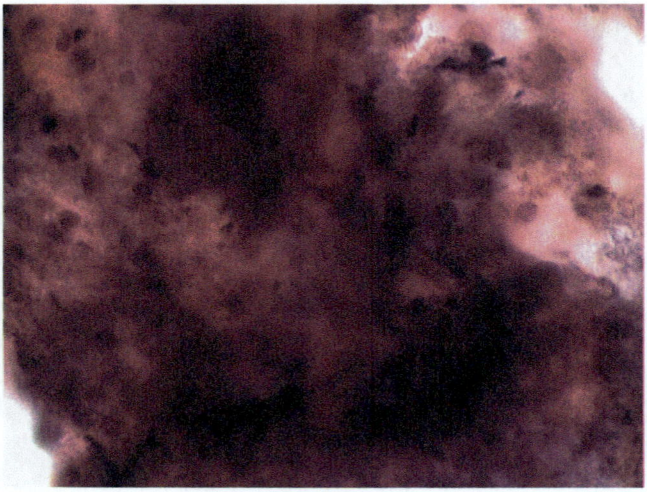

Fig. 10.3 Obscuring of cellular material: Specimen was uninterpretable due to complete obscuring by bacteria-laden oral mucus

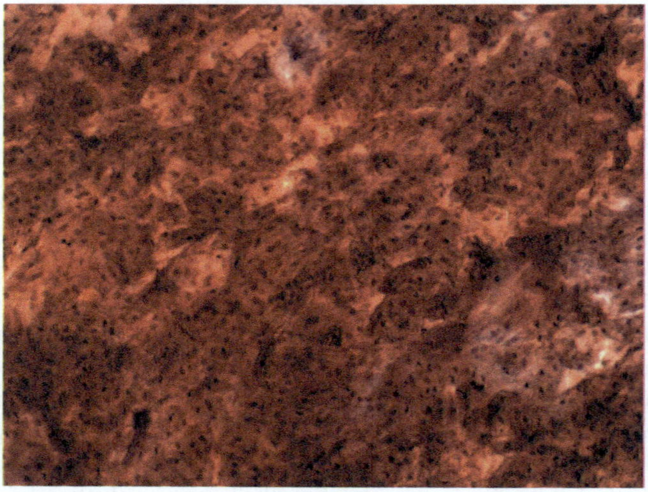

Fig. 10.4 Improper smear technique: Poor distribution of cellular material resulted in an excessively thick smear, precluding interpretation of individual cells

False negatives:

- Failure to recognize rare cancerous/precancerous cells on microscopy in the background of a large number of exfoliated normal cells that vastly outnumber dysplastic cells (Fig. 10.8).

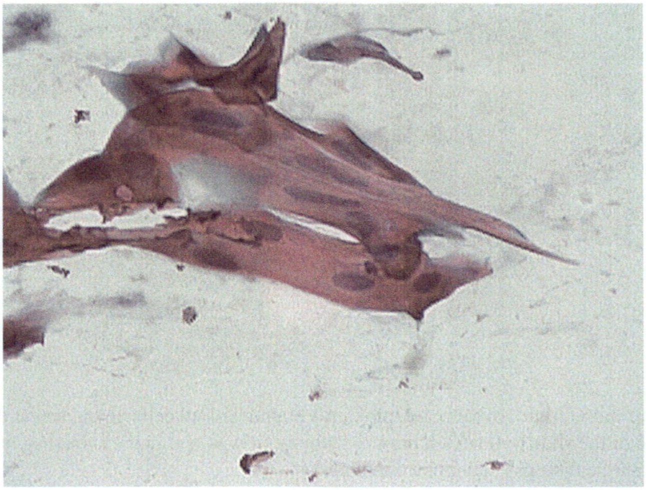

Fig. 10.5 Improper smear technique: "Smearing" artifact caused by excessively heavy-handed brush to slide transfer with resulting cellular distortion

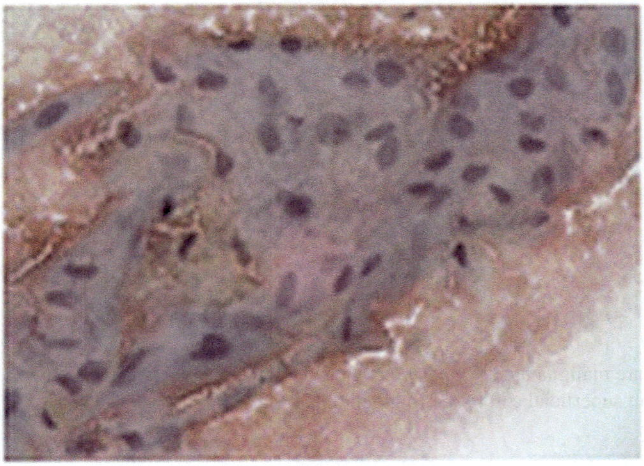

Fig. 10.6 Air drying artifact: Loss of nuclear chromatin detail and cytoplasmic differentiation

- The deceptively bland cytology of verrucous carcinoma, especially those examples with superimposed inflammatory changes may mislead an inexperienced cytopathologist. Verrucous carcinoma of the oral cavity, akin to that in the uterine cervix is rare. The cytology of this lesion mirrors its bland histology. The cytologic features of verrucous carcinoma in the uterine cervix include atypical polygonal and spindle cells with abundant, keratinizing cytoplasm, atypical squamous cells with pearl formation, and frequent,

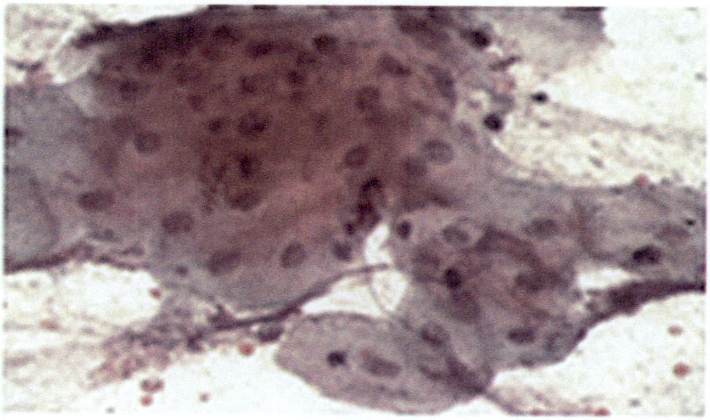

Fig. 10.7 Pap stain failure: In this case, pink gray staining of all cells on the smear due to inadvertent exposure of the slide to formalin prior to staining (it was sent in the same bag with an improperly secured surgical biopsy specimen container)

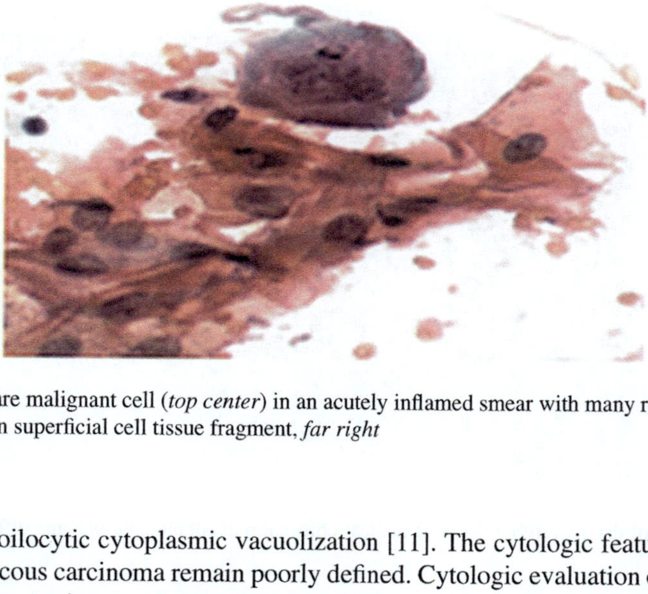

Fig. 10.8 Rare malignant cell (*top center*) in an acutely inflamed smear with many reactive cells. Note hypha in superficial cell tissue fragment, *far right*

nonkoilocytic cytoplasmic vacuolization [11]. The cytologic features of oral verrucous carcinoma remain poorly defined. Cytologic evaluation of oral verrucous carcinoma may reveal only keratinization of the cytoplasm and cytoplasmic vacuolization (Figs. 10.9a and 10.9b).

- Some well differentiated squamous cell carcinomas may show very subtle changes and may be falsely reported as dysplasias [10].

False positives:

- Reactive atypia secondary to infection or inflammation may be reported as malignancy, especially if appropriate clues are not recognized (Fig. 10.10).
- Dysplastic changes may sometimes be reported as malignant.

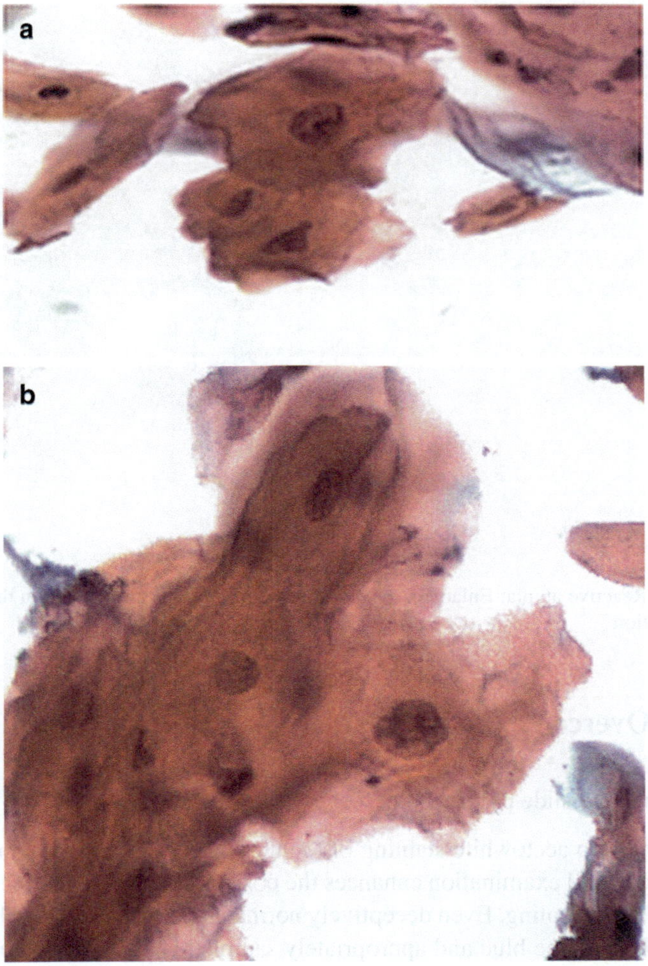

Fig. 10.9 (**a** and **b**) Verrucous carcinoma: Increased cytoplasmic keratinization and nuclear enlargement are the only clues; in an inflammatory background these could easily be misinterpreted as reactive. The complete absence of background inflammation leads to properly flagging this case as abnormal

5. "*Pathologic processes requiring interpretation of architectural features for identification*" Conclusions about the architectural features of a lesion cannot be made from evaluation of a cytology specimen as:
   (a) The relationship of the cells to one another can not be studied as they can in biopsy specimens.
   (b) Often, only individual cells are observed so that all the pathognomic features of the disease may not be present [12].

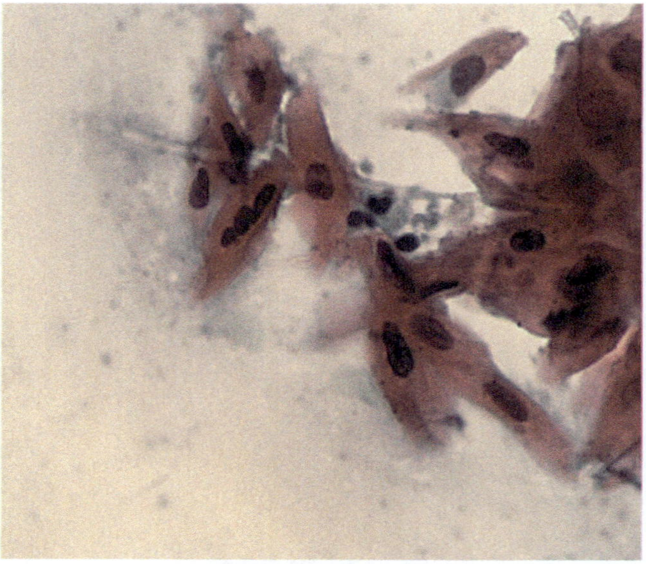

Fig. 10.10 Reactive atypia: Enlarged, hyperchromatic, superficial cell nuclei, in this case due to fungal infection

How to Overcome the Pitfalls?

1. Sampling and slide preparation:
   (a) Similar to acetowhite staining of the uterine cervix, Toluidine blue staining during oral examination enhances the possibility of selecting the appropriate site for sampling. Even deceptively normal appearing areas can be identified with toluidine blue and appropriately sampled [10]. Toluidine blue has also proved useful for assessing the status of margins around oral cancer at the time of resection [13]. Although toluidine blue staining provide valuable assistance in the identification of oral cancers, it should not be viewed as a substitute for biopsy as a negative test does not preclude the presence of dysplasia or even oral cancer.
   (b) Sampling of ulcers should focus on the edges of the lesion as avoidance of the center is most likely to yield viable cells without abundant obscuring necrotic debris, enhancing the possibility of obtaining and identifying diagnostic cells.
   (c) If there is exudate, debris, or other non-viable or non-cellular material on the surface of a lesion, an effort should be made to remove it before sampling to avoid contamination and false negative results.
   (d) Full thickness sampling (indicated by pin point bleeding) should be done so as to include the basal layer where the dysplastic changes often first appear. Use of oral brushes have overcome the problem of full thickness sampling to

a great extent [14]. The accuracy of the brush test has been the subject of many published studies. In every study in which an oral lesion was simultaneously tested with both a brush biopsy and scalpel biopsy, this test has been shown to have a sensitivity and specificity well over 90% [15].

(e) Good quality smears should be prepared with transfer of all of the cellular material on to the slide, proper spreading and distribution of cellular material, and optimal fixation and staining. Use of liquid based cytology has improved the sampling procedure and has minimized the pitfalls associated with conventional smear preparations. By decreasing the mucus, inflammatory components, and blood in a preparation, more homogenous samples are obtained [16–19]. Another advantage of liquid based cytology is that remaining cells in the collection fluid can be used for additional tests [20–22].

It should be noted, however, that liquid based techniques were designed for exfoliative cytology samples and they do not reliably preserve epithelial tissue fragments and the three-dimensional "microbiopsies" collected by a brush biopsy sample, which may inhibit proper microscopic evaluation of the specimen [23].

2. Microscopy:

(a) Adequate training of cytopathologists is a must [24]. They should be well versed with the pathologic findings of the various lesions of the oral cavity and aware of the various pitfalls.

(b) The reporting cytopathologist should be provided with all the clinical information pertaining to the lesion. It is of critical value, especially when differentiating reactive atypia from neoplasia and dysplasia from well differentiated squamous cell carcinoma. A characteristic clinical history and appearance may be essential for identification of verrucous carcinoma which is notoriously difficult to diagnose on cytology.

(c) The reporting cytopathologist should always perform a careful and conscientious search for potentially neoplastic changes as this may enable the clinician to provide timely treatment to the patient, lessening the morbidity and mortality.

References

1. Jones AC, Pink FE, Sandow PL, Stewart CM, Migliorati CA, Baughman RA. The Cytobrush Plus cell collector in oral cytology. Oral Surg Oral Med Oral Pathol. 1994;77:95–9.
2. Remmerbach TW, Meyer-Ebrecht D, Aach T, et al. Toward a multimodal cell analysis of brush biopsies for the early detection of oral cancer. Cancer Cytopathol. 2009;117:228–35.
3. Ogden GR. The future role for oral exfoliative cytology – bleak or bright? Oral Oncol. 1997;33:2–4.
4. Dabelsteen E, Roed-Petersen B, Smith CJ, Pindborg JJ. The limitations of exfoliative cytology for detection of epithelial atypia in oral leukoplakias. Br J Cancer. 1971;25:21–4.
5. Folsom TC, White CP, Bromer L, Canby HF, Garrington GE. Oral exfoliative study. Review of the literature and report of a 3 year study. Oral Surg Oral Med Oral Pathol. 1972;33:61–74.

6. From exfoliative cytology to oral brush biopsy: an advance in the early detection of oral pre-cancers and cancers. http://oralcancerfoundation.org/products/detailed_brush_cytology.htm. Accessed 1 Jan 2012.
7. Diniz-Freitas M, Garcia-Garcia A, Crespo-Abelleira A, Martins-Carneiro JL, Gandara-Rey JM. Applications of exfoliative cytology in the diagnosis of oral cancer. Med Oral. 2004;9:355–61.
8. Navone R, Pentenero M, Rostan I, et al. Oral potentially malignant lesions: first-level micro-histological diagnosis from tissue fragments sampled in liquid-based diagnostic cytology. J Oral Pathol. 2008;37:358–63.
9. Mehrotra R, Hullmann M, Smeets R, Reichert TE, Driemel O. Oral cytology revisited. J Oral Pathol Med. 2009;38:161–6.
10. Divani S, Exarhou M, et al. Advantages and difficulties of brush cytology in the identification of early oral cancer. Arch Oncol. 2009;17:11–2.
11. Pantanowitz L, Upton MP, Wang HH, Nasser I. Cytomorphology of verrucous carcinoma of the cervix. A case report. Acta Cytol. 2003;47(6):1050–4.
12. Kujan O, Desai M, Sargent A, Bailey A, et al. Potential applications of oral brush cytology with liquid based technology: results from a cohort of normal oral mucosa. Oral Oncol. 2006;42:810–8.
13. Epstein JB, Güneri P. The adjunctive role of toluidine blue in detection of oral premalignant and malignant lesions. Curr Opin Otolaryngol Head Neck Surg. 2009;17(2):79–87.
14. Mehrotra R, Gupta G, Singh M, Ibrahim R. Application of cytology and molecular biology in diagnosing premalignant or malignant oral lesions. Mol Cancer. 2006;5:11–8.
15. Scheifele C, Schmidt-Westhausen AM, Dietrich T, Reichart A. The sensitivity and specificity of the oral CDx technique: evaluation of 103 cases. Oral Oncol. 2004;40:824–8.
16. Navone R, Burlo P, Pich A, Pentenero M, et al. The impact of liquid based oral cytology the diagnosis of oral squamous dysplasia and carcinoma. Cytopathology. 2007;18:356–60.
17. Kahn MA. Oral exfoliative cytology procedures: conventional, brush biopsy and Thin Prep. J Tenn Dent Assoc. 2001;81:17–20.
18. Bernstein ML, Miller RL. Oral exfoliative cytology. J Am Dent Assoc. 1978;96:625–9.
19. Hayama FH, Motta AC, Silva-Ade P, Migliari DA. Liquid based preparations versus conventional cytology: specimen adequacy and diagnostic agreement in oral lesions. Med Oral Patol Oral Cir Bucal. 2005;10:115–22.
20. Yoshida T, Fukuda T, Sano T, Kanuma T, Owada N, Nakajima T. Usefulness of liquid based cytology specimens for the immunocytochemical study of p16 expression and human papillomavirus testing: a comparative study using simultaneously sampled histology materials. Cancer. 2004;102:100–8.
21. Lorenzato M, Bory JP, Cucherousset J, et al. Usefulness of DNA ploidy measurement on liquid-based smears showing conflicting results between cytology and high risk human papillomavirus typing. Am J Clin Pathol. 2002;118:708–13.
22. Wojcik EM, Saraga SA, Jin JK, Hendricks JB. Application of laser scanning cytometry for evaluation of DNA ploidy in routine cytologic specimens. Diagn Cytopathol. 2001;24:200–5.
23. Hullmann M, Reichert TE, Dahse R, et al. Orale Zytologie: Historische Entwicklung, aktueller Stand und Ausblick. Mund Kiefer Gesichtschir. 2007;11:01–9.
24. Gologan O, Hunt JL. Potential diagnostic use of p16INK4A, a new marker that correlates with dysplasia in oral squamoproliferative lesions. Am J Surg Pathol. 2005;29:792–6.

Chapter 11
The Way Ahead: Overview of Present Day Use with Areas for Future Research

Ravi Mehrotra

The prognosis for patients with oral squamous cell carcinoma remains poor in spite of advances in therapy of many other cancers. Early diagnosis and treatment remains the key to improved patient survival. There is an urgent need to devise critical diagnostic tools for the early detection of oral potentially malignant as well as malignant lesions that are practical, noninvasive and can be easily performed in an out-patient setting [1].

The clinician's challenge is to differentiate cancerous lesions from a multitude of other red, white, or ulcerated lesions that also occur in the oral cavity. Most oral lesions are benign, but many have an appearance that may be confused with a malignant lesion, and some previously considered benign are now classified premalignant—because they have been statistically correlated with subsequent malignant changes. Conversely, some malignant lesions seen at a very early stage, may be mistaken for a benign entity. Any oral lesion that does not regress spontaneously or respond to the usual therapeutic measures should be considered potentially malignant until histologically shown to be benign on investigation. A period of 2–3 weeks is considered an appropriate period of time to evaluate the response of a lesion.

Numerous potentially malignant oral lesions, primarily leukoplakia (especially the speckled variety) and erythroplakia, occur frequently in adults (Figs. 11.1 and 11.2). Developing useful approaches to their prevention, increasing the accuracy of diagnosis, discovering reliable biologic markers for these lesions, and improving their management will all further the enviable goal of oral cancer control.

However, in spite of all attempts to prevent them, oral cancers continue to occur. Therefore, early diagnosis combined with adequate treatment is critical for reducing the substantial morbidity and mortality associated with this disease, which has not improved significantly over the last so many years, in spite of some remarkable

R. Mehrotra (✉)
Institute of Cytology and Preventive Oncology (ICPO), I-7, Sector - 39, Noida - 201301, Uttar Pradesh, India
e-mail: rm8509@gmail.com

R. Mehrotra (ed.), *Oral Cytology: A Concise Guide*, DOI 10.1007/978-1-4614-5221-8_11,

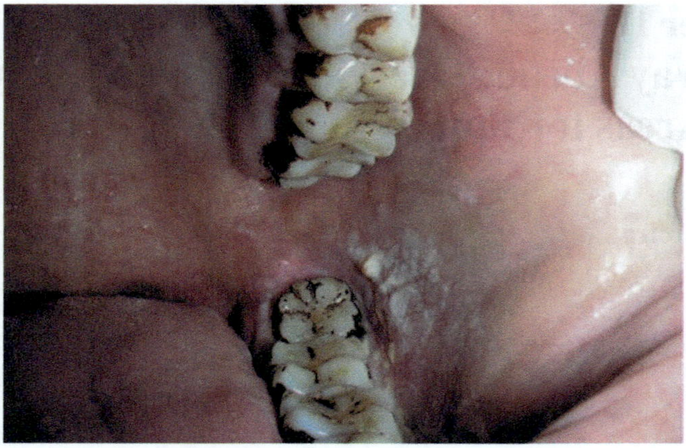

Fig. 11.1 Clinical picture of a patient with leukoplakia (Mehrotra R, Thomas S, Nair P, Pandya S, Singh M, Nigam NS, Shukla P. Prevalence of oral soft tissue lesions in Vidisha. BMC Res Notes 2010; 3: 23)

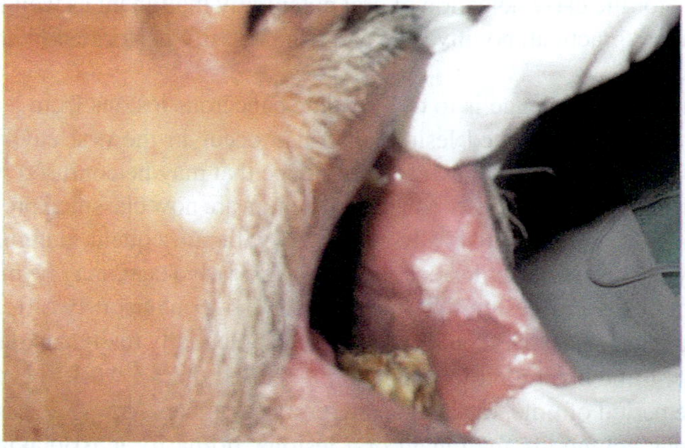

Fig. 11.2 Clinical picture of a patient with speckled leukoplakia (Mehrotra R, Thomas S, Nair P, Pandya S, Singh M, Nigam NS, Shukla P. Prevalence of oral soft tissue lesions in Vidisha. BMC Res Notes 2010; 3: 23)

advances in outcome of therapy of many other malignancies—some of which had similarly dismal prognosis not too long back.

If there is a delay in or contraindication to biopsy, exfoliative cytology (cell scrapings) may serve as an adjunct to clinical diagnosis, as it enables a more extensive screening and at the same time, provides cytological material. However, cytologic smears are used infrequently and, so far, patients are not treated on the basis of cytologic findings alone. Smears are most helpful in differentiating inflammatory conditions, especially Candidiasis, from dysplastic or neoplastic surface lesions. In addition, cytology may be helpful in detecting field changes in oral cancer, especially if this method is used in conjunction with vital staining. Cytology may also be helpful when ulcerations following radiation are suspicious and biopsy is delayed [2].

Fine needle aspiration biopsy of subsurface head and neck masses is also an accepted diagnostic test and its usage has increased in popularity over the past few years. This technique is extremely useful in evaluating clinically suspicious changes involving salivary glands and lymph nodes. It expedites diagnosis/staging and may, at times, obviate the need of an incisional or excisional biopsy. When used by a skilled clinician, fine needle aspiration can often be the best way to establish a definitive diagnosis. It is also valuable in following up patients with a previous malignancy, as well as, where the possibility of viral etiology of an oropharyngeal malignancy is considered [3].

Approaches to Early Detection of Dysplasia and Oral Cancer

There are two approaches in the early detection of oral dysplasia and cancer: (1) oral cancer screening programs that identify asymptomatic patients with suspicious lesions and (2) employing specific diagnostic tools to identify dysplasia and early oral cancers in asymptomatic patients with an oral abnormality. The benefits and limitations of these approaches will be addressed in this chapter.

Oral Cancer Screening

Screening for oral cancer entails searching for oral precancerous and cancerous lesions, typically before symptoms occur. A number of established cancer screening programs for a variety of malignancies have been shown to significantly reduce patient morbidity and mortality—including the Papanicolaou test for cervical cancer and mammography for breast cancer. Oral cancer screening is fraught with problems including the fact that approximately 5–15% of the general population may have an oral mucosal lesion. The classic clinical presentation of a premalignant lesion or malignancy includes a red spot, white spot or persistent ulcer. However, only a small percentage of these types of lesions are malignant and an oral examination unfortunately often cannot discriminate between lesions that are potentially dangerous from condtions that are benign. Several publications have demonstrated that visual oral cancer screening has limited value as a method for detecting precancerous or early cancerous lesions. In the only randomized controlled oral cancer screening trial conducted in India and involving over 130,000 individuals, the authors concluded that visual examination was useful as a method of screening for oral cancer only in high risk cases like chronic smokers or alcoholics [4]. A recent Cochrane review on this subject failed to find any evidence to confirm or refute the usefulness of visual screening for oral malignancy [5]. The review concluded that "although there is evidence that a visual examination as part of a population based screening program reduced the mortality rate of oral cancer in high-risk individuals, whilst producing a stage shift and improvement in survival rates across the population as a whole, the evidence is limited to one study and is associated with a high risk of bias".

Diagnostic Tests

Oral squamous cell carcinoma (OSCC) is almost always preceded by a visible precancerous lesion-dysplasia. As highlighted by the American Dental Association, "Identifying white and red spots that show dysplasia and removing them before they become cancer has proved to be one of the most effective methods for reducing the incidence and mortality of cancer" [6]. Malignant transformation of dysplasia, which is quite unpredictable, occurs over years—during which time the lesion can be treated—potentially preventing oral cancer from developing. Oral precancerous lesions may also occasionally regress if the healthcare professional motivates the patient to reduce the risk factors including elimination of carcinogens including tobacco and alcohol [7].

The practice of not properly evaluating all suspicious lesions, that is, lesions without a specific etiology such as trauma or infection, invariably results in delay of the correct diagnosis, limiting treatment options. This may be attributed to lack of awareness about these lesions by dentists, head and neck surgeons and other primary care providers, non-compliance of patients maximally at risk, inexperience and lack of familiarity with biopsy techniques as well as dearth of minimally invasive and painless reliable diagnostic techniques.

Cytological Techniques

During the last few decades, interest in the usage of oral cytology has undergone a resurgence. However, in contrast to the sampling of cells of the uterine cervix, analysis of surface epithelial cells of the oral cavity and oropharynx by standard exfoliative cytology is not widespread. The shape of the oral cavity makes it impossible to examine the complete mucosal surface, specially the posterior pharynx. In addition, without loss of minimal invasiveness, it was not possible to access the deeper cell layers of the oral cavity with conventional exfoliative cytology [8]. Thus conventional methods of cell sampling have not gained acceptance in the medical community. On the other hand, Dolens et al. from São Paulo, in a very recent meta-analysis performed according to Preferred Reporting Items for Systematic Reviews and Meta-Analyses guidelines, reported that the I-square test for conventional cytology showed a sensitivity of 80.2% and specificity of 96.7%. They evaluated 80 relevant articles in the literature between 1967 and 2010, and 14 of which were included in this study. The area under the curve was 0.9901 with an ideal of 1. The authors concluded that cytology has good sensitivity and specificity for the diagnosis of oral lesions and allowed the use of other associated techniques, such as DNA analysis, that may improve the accuracy of cytology [9]. The initial wave of enthusiasm for the technique of the 1970s and 1980s has now given way to cautious optimism after employment of modern techniques involving novel sampling instruments as well as automated image analysis. In an attempt to localize the optimal site for brushing an abnormality, Gupta et al. have combined conventional oral brush biopsy with the application of toluidine blue [10].

Brush Biopsy

During the 1980s, a brush was introduced for cervical smears in gynecological lesions and was later modified for oral smears too. This technique demonstrated better cell spreading on objective slides compared with smears obtained by using the conventional wooden spatula as well as an improvement in the cellular adequacy of the smears. Unlike exfoliative cytology, the brush biopsy collects cells from the full thickness of the oral epithelium. The brush biopsy is a chair-side, easy to perform, painless test that can be used to evaluate any suspicious lesion including common small white and red oral lesions to rule out dysplasia. Since most oral lesions are benign, majority of the test results are likely to be benign. Approximately 10% of all cases usually turn out to be abnormal. Based upon the findings, the laboratory provides specific guidance on these abnormal cases sometimes recommending scalpel biopsy, retesting or observation.

The accuracy of the brush test has been the subject of many published studies. In every study in which an oral lesion was simultaneously tested with both a brush biopsy and scalpel biopsy, this test has been shown to have a sensitivity and specificity of well over 90% [11–14].

Discrepancies of brush test and scalpel biopsy results have been reported anecdotally and have incorrectly been labeled brush "false negatives." Unfortunately, these anecdotes have been quoted repeatedly in the literature despite the fact that they have no validity at all. In all probability, these discrepant results were all from cases where the scalpel biopsy was performed months after the brush biopsy. Within a given oral lesion, dysplasia may be multifocal and unless the two biopsies happen to sample the same part of the dysplastic lesion, the results may well be discrepant. Furthermore, the biologic nature of a lesion may change over time as benign lesions may become dysplastic and dysplasia may also regress. Most importantly, the histologic diagnosis of dysplasia is not easily reproduced amongst oral pathologists and therefore a discrepant result between brush biopsy and scalpel biopsy may in fact even represent a false negative or false positive scalpel biopsy result. Therefore, when comparisons are made between any two biopsy techniques (i.e. brush biopsy vs. scalpel biopsy or scalpel biopsy vs. scalpel biopsy) the only valid studies are those which compare the results of both biopsies performed at the same time and from the same portion of the suspicious lesion. A wide variety of benign and dysplastic changes are observed in the oral brush slides. Malignant cells showing abnormalities like binucleation, hyperchromasia and hyperkeratinization can also be seen (Figs. 11.3–11.7).

A frequent criticism of the brush test has been that Class II or minimally suspicious lesions have not been simultaneously tested both by cytologic and scalpel biopsy examination. Addressing these issues, the authors' group performed oral brush and

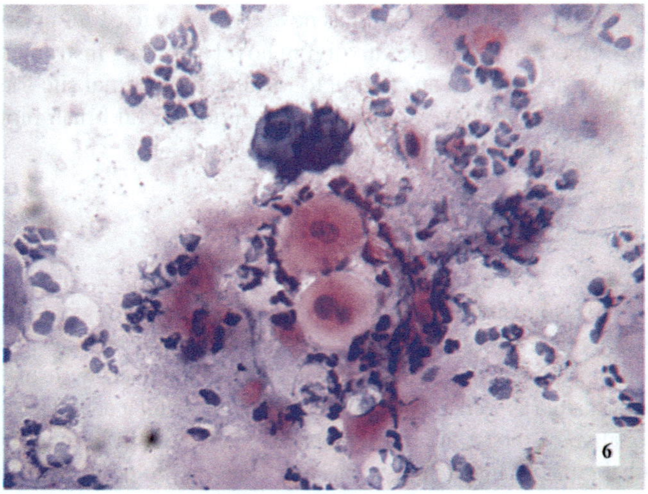

Fig. 11.3 Photomicrograph of an oral brush biopsy specimen from a patient of squamous cell carcinoma of the buccal mucosa showing a binucleated cell with evidence of intracellular and extracellular keratinization in an inflammatory background. (H & E ×400) (Mehrotra R, Gupta A, Singh M, Ibrahim R. Application of cytology in diagnosing premalignant or malignant oral lesions. Mol Cancer 2006; 5: 1)

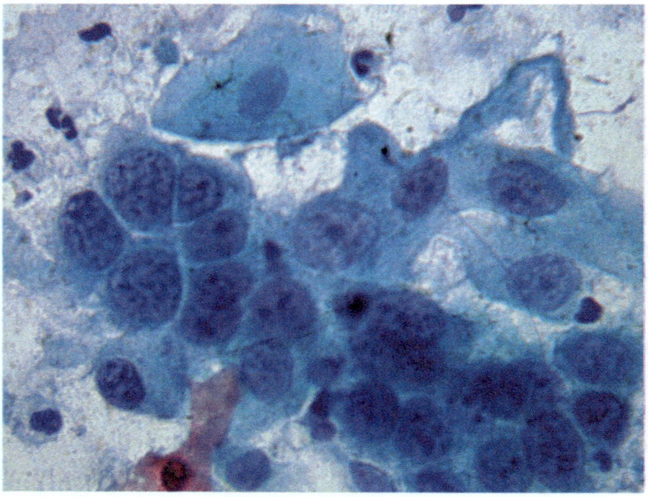

Fig. 11.4 Photomicrograph of an oral brush biopsy specimen from a patient of squamous cell carcinoma of the buccal mucosa with high nucleo-cytoplasmic ratio marked atypia, and coarsely granular chromatin in a necrotic background. (Modified Pap ×1,000) (Mehrotra R, Gupta A, Singh M, Ibrahim R. Application of cytology in diagnosing premalignant or malignant oral lesions. Mol Cancer 2006; 5: 1)

scalpel biopsies on 85 consecutive patients presenting with an oral lesion deemed to be minimally suspicious by clinical examination (Figs. 11.8 and 11.9) and the results were compared. In case of any discrepancy between the cytologic and histopathological

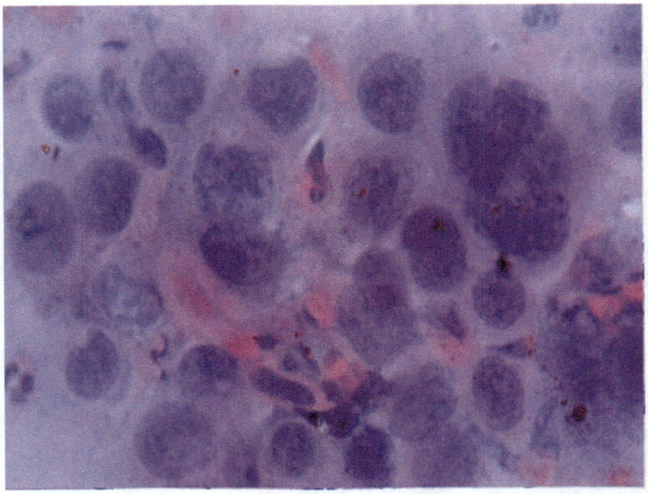

Fig. 11.5 Photomicrograph of an oral brush biopsy specimen from a patient of squamous cell carcinoma of buccal mucosa with high nucleo-cytoplasmic ratio coarsely granular chromatin and a multinucleated cell showing evidence of vascular invasion. (H&E ×1,000) (Mehrotra R, Gupta A, Singh M, Ibrahim R. Application of cytology in diagnosing premalignant or malignant oral lesions. Mol Cancer 2006; 5: 1)

findings, the presence of a brush defect in the biopsy material confirmed that the sample has been taken from the same area (Fig. 11.10). Of 79 patients with adequate brush samples with matching scalpel biopsies, 27 revealed histopathological evidence of dysplasia or carcinoma, 26 of which were independently identified with the oral brush biopsy. The positive predictive value of an abnormal oral brush biopsy was 84% and the negative predictive value was 98%. This study conclusively provided proof that this is an accurate test in identifying oral premalignant and malignant lesions, even if minimally suspicious. The test was found to be especially beneficial when used on lesions that appear clinically benign for identifying early stage cancers and dysplasia—the lesions for which therapy is most effective. It was concluded that as an adjunct to oral examination, its use has the potential to reduce the poor mortality rate associated with oral malignancies [14].

Fluorescence

Candida is a highly underdiagnosed fungal infection common among elderly patients, denture wearers, patients with impaired salivary gland function, medicated patients, diets high in carbohydrates, smokers, diabetics, Cushing's syndrome, oral malignancies, and in immunodeficiency diseases such as HIV infection. Literature search reveals incidence rates ranging from 20% to 75% [15]. A recent study demonstrated that Papanicolaou stained oral squamous cells and Candida autofluoresce bright green under autofluorescence microscopy. The authors concluded that orientation of

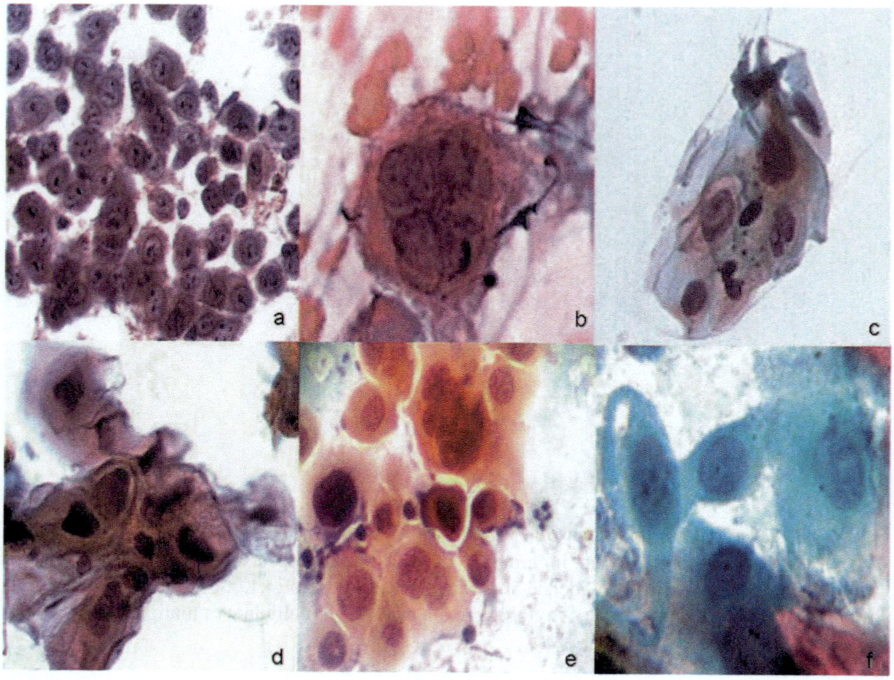

Fig. 11.6 Panorama of cellular abnormalities. (**a**) Pemphigus (Papanicolaou, 3100). (**b**) Giant cell in a patient with herpes simplex virus infection (Papanicolaou, 3100). (**c**) Post radiation nucleomegaly (Papanicolaou, 3100). (**d**) Atypical squamous cells consistent with dysplasia (Papanicolaou, 3100). (**e**) Pleomorphism and hyperchromasia in an oral malignancy (Papanicolaou, 3100). (**f**) Tadpole cell in oral malignancy (Papanicolaou, 3100) [8]

the Candida hyphae and autofluorescing squamous cells affected screening results. Hyphae otherwise undetected under light microscopy may be identified under autofluorescence microscopy, and vice versa. PAS stained oral cytology viewed with normal light microscopy remains the gold standard with regard to identifying oral candidiasis or the carrier state [16]. This topic has been covered in more detail in Chap. 4.

Ploidy Examination

DNA ploidy status has been investigated to determine the malignant potential of cells. After staining with Feulgen dye, the cytologic samples are compared with a reference group of cells. A computer-assisted analysis has been recently designed to identify deviations of cellular DNA content. Genomic instability contributes towards cancer development, and abnormal DNA content may distinguish the dysplastic lesions that might progress to cancer [17]. Several studies confirm the usefulness of

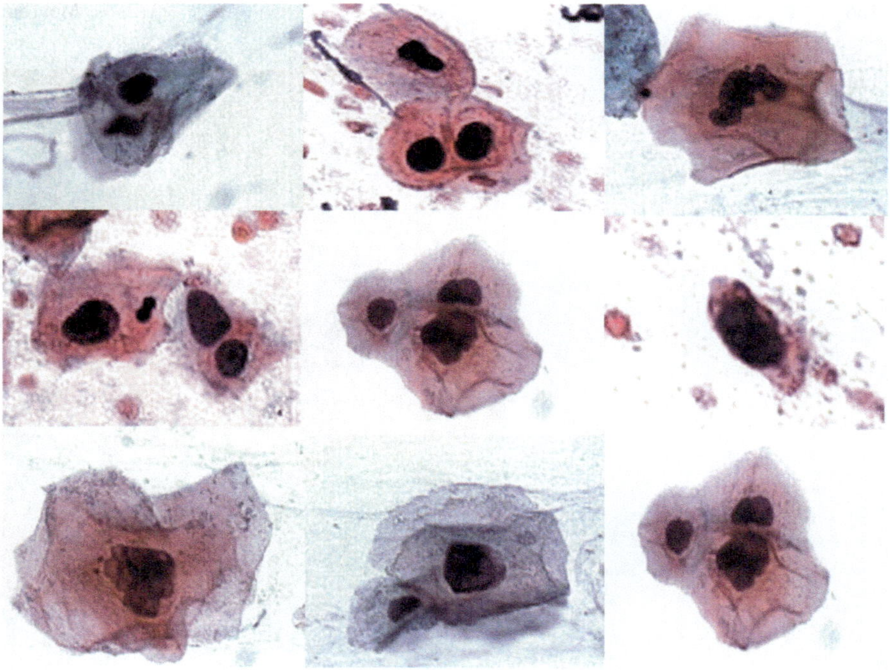

Fig. 11.7 Gallery of atypical and malignant cells identified from a brush biopsy specimen with the aid of a highly specialized neural network-based image-processing system. (Pap ×1,000) [14]

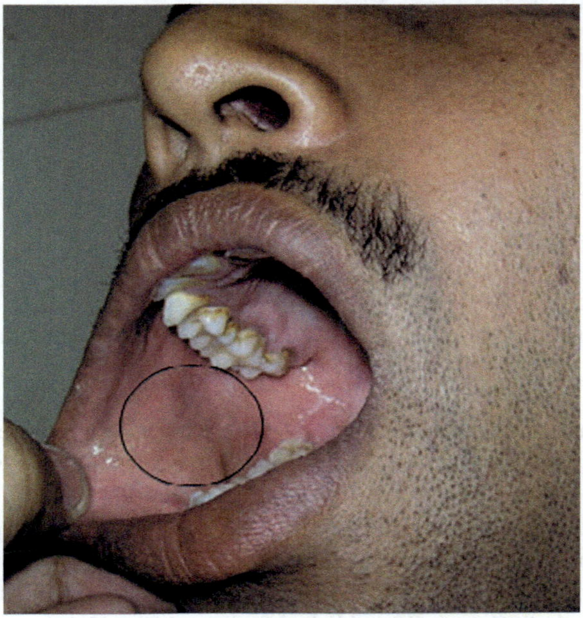

Fig. 11.8 Example of a clinically minimally suspicious Class II lesion [14]

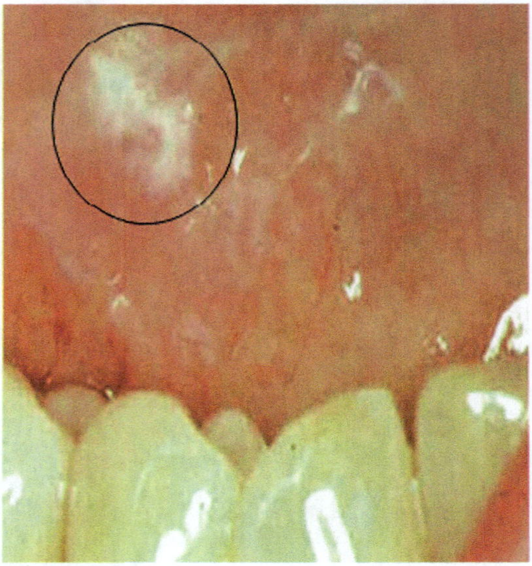

Fig. 11.9 Another example of a clinically minimally suspicious Class II lesion [14]

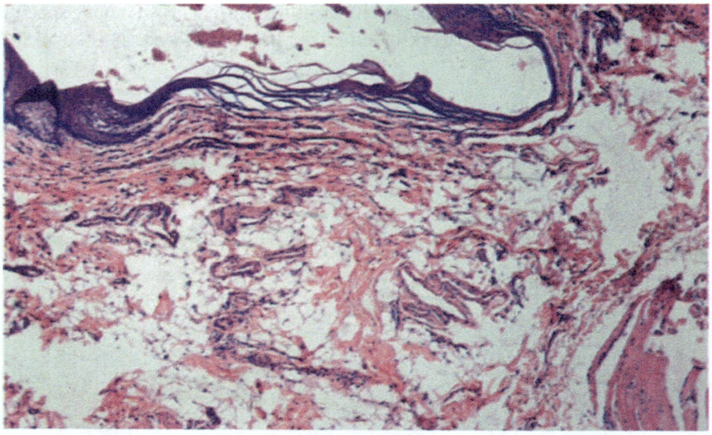

Fig. 11.10 Histopathologic specimen demonstrating the oral biopsy defect sampling the entire thickness of the epithelium. (H &E ×100) [14]

DNA ploidy analysis as an adjunct to conventional cytology assessment of cytobrush samples for detection of oral cancer [17–20]. An increase in sensitivity and specificity of oral brush biopsy to 100% has been reported [19, 21]. In an on-going study, the author studied 65 patients who underwent simultaneous ploidy analysis and scalpel biopsy, and a reproducible correlation was found between abnormal ploidy status and dysplasia/malignancy—yielding sensitivity and specificity rates of approximately 90% each (Unpublished findings—Fig. 11.11).

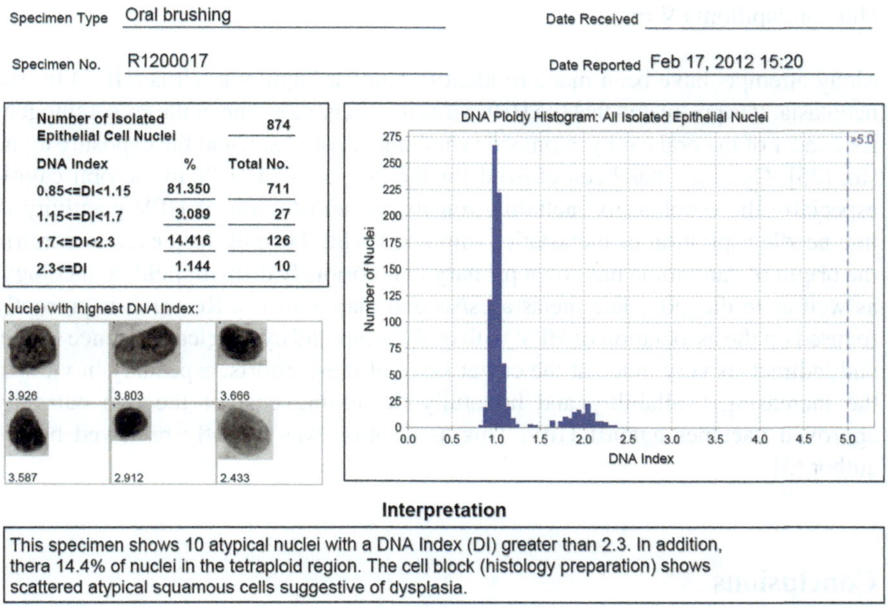

Specimen Type Oral brushing

Date Received

Specimen No. R1200017

Date Reported Feb 17, 2012 15:20

Number of Isolated Epithelial Cell Nuclei		874
DNA Index	%	Total No.
0.85<=DI<1.15	81.350	711
1.15<=DI<1.7	3.089	27
1.7<=DI<2.3	14.416	126
2.3<=DI	1.144	10

Nuclei with highest DNA Index:

Interpretation

This specimen shows 10 atypical nuclei with a DNA Index (DI) greater than 2.3. In addition, thera 14.4% of nuclei in the tetraploid region. The cell block (histology preparation) shows scattered atypical squamous cells suggestive of dysplasia.

Fig. 11.11 Abnormal DNA ploidy from an oral brushing Courtesy: Oral Advance®, Vancouver, BC, Canada

Nanochip-Based Systems

In a recent pilot study, Weigum et al. [22] used a single nano-bio-chip platform for molecular and morphologic analysis in oral exfoliative cytology to enhance the role and utility of oral cytology in clinical diagnostics. The integration of the nano-bio-chip sensor system for concurrent and quantitative analysis of cellular biomarkers and cytomorphology has been studied in 41 patients and 11 controls for multifunctional cytoanalysis. They found six parameters to be significantly altered in OSCC cytospecimens versus healthy mucosa, including (a) nuclear area, (b) nuclear diameter, (c) cellular area, (d) cellular diameter, (e) nuclear-to-cytoplasmic ratio, and (f) EGFR biomarker immunolabeling. The nuclear area, nuclear diameter, nuclear-to-cytoplasmic ratio, and EGFR expression were also found to be significantly altered in oral lesions with diagnosed dysplasia, supporting the use of these markers as diagnostic indicators of early cancer development and premalignancy. These findings are in line with earlier reports by Ramaesh and Ratanatunga [24], identifying significant changes in cellular and nuclear morphology. Although it's early days yet, this methodology may well be the way of the future and needs exploring.

Human Papilloma Virus

Many attempts have been made to identify Human Papilloma virus (HPV) in oral neoplasia. It is postulated that the HPV virus may behave as one of the co-carcinogens for cancer of the oral cavity, alongside smoking, alcoholism, and the exposure to the sun [25]. Cytology has been utilized for the diagnosis of HPV in the oral cavity, especially the oropharynx including tonsils. Demonstration of HPV positivity in fine needle aspiration of metastatic lymph nodes has been utilized even to confirm the origin of carcinoma unknown primary (a notoriously difficult field in oncology) as well as to diagnose late metastases/second malignancies. Research is presently focused on the association of HPV with oral lesions and cytological evidence (direct and indirect) is very much at the center stage of these efforts, especially in view of the increasing availability and hopefully decreasing cost of the two currently approved vaccines against HPV. This association was recently reviewed by the author [3].

Conclusions

Early detection of OSCCs not only increases the survival rate but also reduces the need for disfiguring treatment. Unfortunately, early detection of oral cancerous lesions has proved difficult because as many as 50% of the patients have regional or distant metastases at the time of diagnosis. The malignant transformation at the beginning of carcinogenesis affects only few cells—long before small parts of tissue are involved. Thus, cytologic examination should be a suitable method to elucidate the nature of suspicious oral lesions—even earlier than histology. Future studies on oral cytology should prove its application on small doubtful lesions. It is necessary to introduce novel adjunctive techniques to cytologic diagnosis for the monitoring of potentially malignant lesions to prevent oral malignancy in its earliest stages of development.

References

1. Mehrotra R, Gupta DK. Exciting new advances in oral cancer diagnosis: avenues to early detection. Head Neck Oncol. 2011;3:33.
2. Mehrotra R, Madhu, Singh M. Serial scrape smear cytology of radiation response in normal and malignant oral cells. Indian J Pathol Microbiol. 2004;47:497–502.
3. Mehrotra R, Sharma N, Umudum H, Ceyhan K, Rezanko T. The role of cytopathology in diagnosing HPV induced oropharyngeal lesions. Diagn Cytopathol. 2012. doi:10.1002/dc.21756.
4. Sankaranarayanan R, Ramadas K, Thomas G, Muwonge R, Thara S, Mathew B, Rajan B, Trivandrum Oral Cancer Screening Study Group. Effect of screening on oral cancer mortality in Kerala, India: a cluster-randomised controlled trial. Lancet. 2005;365(9475):1927–33.

5. Brocklehurst P, Kujan O, Glenny AM, Oliver R, Sloan P, Ogden G, Shepherd S. Screening programmes for the early detection and prevention of oral cancer. Cochrane Database Syst Rev. 2010 (11):CD004150.
6. http://www.ada.org/2607.aspxLast. Accessed 1 Mar 2012.
7. Burzynski NJ, Firriolo FJ, Butters JM, Sorrell CL. Evaluation of oral cancer screening. J Cancer Educ. 1997;12(2):95–9.
8. Mehrotra R. The role of cytology in oral lesions: a review of recent improvements. Diagn Cytopathol. 2012;40:73–83.
9. Dolens EDS, Nakai FVD, Parizi JL, Nai GA. Cytopathology: a useful technique for diagnosing oral lesions? A systematic literature review. Diagn Cytopathol. 2012. Epub ahead of print.
10. Gupta A, Singh M, Ibrahim R, Mehrotra R. Utility of toluidine blue and oral brush biopsy in oral precancerous lesions and squamous cell carcinoma. Acta Cytol. 2007;51:788–94.
11. Mehrotra R, Hullmann M, Smeets R, Reichert TE, Driemel O: Oral cytology revisited. J Oral Pathol Med. 2009;38(2):161–166.
12. Sciubba JJ. Improving detection of precancerous and cancerous oral lesions. Computer-assisted analysis of the oral brush biopsy. J Am Dent Assoc. 1999;130:1445–57.
13. Scheifele C, Schmidt-Westhausen AM, Dietrich T, Reichart A. The sensitivity and specificity of the oral CDx technique: evaluation of 103 cases. Oral Oncol. 2004;40:824–8.
14. Mehrotra R, Mishra S, Singh M, Singh M. The efficacy of oral brush biopsy with computer-assisted analysis in identifying precancerous and cancerous lesions. Head Neck Oncol. 2011;3:39.
15. Adam T, Göbel UB, Graf B. Qualitative and quantitative studies of autofluorescence in fungi. Mycoses. 1998;41:39–46.
16. Titinchi F, Toit JD, Hille JJ, Neethling G. The diagnostic accuracy of autofluorescence microscopy of Pap smears for oral candida hyphae. Int J Oral Maxillofacial Pathol. 2011;2(4):28–33.
17. Bradley G, Odell EW, Raphael S, Ho J, Le LW, Benchimol S, Kamel-Reid S. Abnormal DNA content in oral epithelial dysplasia is associated with increased risk of progression to carcinoma. Br J Cancer. 2010;103(9):1432–42.
18. Maraki D, Becker J, Boecking A. Cytologic and DNA cytometric very early diagnosis of oral cancer. J Oral Pathol Med. 2004;33:398–404.
19. Maraki D, Yalcinkaya S, Pomjanski N, Megahed M, Boecking A, Becker J. Cytologic and DNA-cytometric examination of oral lesions in lichen planus. J Oral Pathol Med. 2006;35(4):227–32.
20. Handschel J, Oz D, Pomjanski N, Depprich R, Ommerborn MA, Braunstein S, Kübler NR, Meyer U, Böcking A. Additional use of DNA-image cytometry improves the assessment of resection margins. J Oral Pathol Med. 2007;36(8):472–5.
21. Remmerbach TW, Mathes SN, Weidenbach H, Hemprich A, Böcking A. Noninvasive brush biopsy as an innovative tool for early detection of oral carcinomas. Mund Kiefer Gesichtschir. 2004;8(4):229–36.
22. Mehrotra R, Vasstrand EN, Ibrahim SO. Recent advances in understanding carcinogenicity of oral squamous cell carcinoma: from basic molecular biology to latest genomic and proteomic findings. Cancer Genomics Proteomics. 2004;1:283–94.
23. Weigum SE, Floriano PN, Redding SW, et al. Nano-Bio-Chip sensor platform for examination of oral exfoliative cytology. Cancer Prev Res. 2010;3:518–28.
24. Ramaesh T, Mendis BR, Ratnatunga N, Thattil RO. Cytomorphometric analysis of squames obtained from normal oral mucosa and lesions of oral leukoplakia and squamous cell carcinoma. J Oral Pathol Med. 1998;27:83–6.
25. Chaudhary AK, Singh M, Sundaram S, Mehrotra R. Role of human papillomavirus and its detection in potentially malignant and malignant head and neck lesions: updated review. Head Neck Oncol. 2009;1:22.

Index

R. Mehrotra (ed.), *Oral Cytology: A Concise Guide*, DOI 10.1007/978-1-4614-5221-8,

M

N

O

9781461452201